LIVING WITH CROH

DR JOAN GOMEZ is Honorary Consulting Psychiatrist to the Chelsea and Westminster Hospital. She was trained at King's College, London, and Westminster Hospital, qualifying MB, BS, and obtained her DPM and MRCPsych in 1973 and 1974 respectively. She was elected a Fellow of the Royal College of Psychiatrists in 1982, and obtained the Diploma in the History of Medicine in 1996 and the Diploma in the Philosophy of Medicine in 1998. She is a Fellow of the Society of Apothecaries and also of the Royal Society of Medicine. She has been engaged in clinical work and research on the interface between psychiatry and physical medicine. Dr Gomez is also the author of four other books published by Sheldon Press: *Coping with Thyroid Problems* (1994), *How to Cope with Bulimia* (1995), *Living with Diabetes* (1995) and *How to Cope with Anaemia* (1998). Her husband was a general practitioner and they have ten children.

Overcoming Common Problems Series

For a full list of titles please contact
Sheldon Press, Marylebone Road, London NW1 4DU

Overcoming Common Problems

Living with Crohn's Disease

Dr Joan Gomez

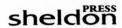

First published in Great Britain in 2000 by
Sheldon Press, SPCK, Marylebone Road, London NW1 4DU

© Joan Gomez 2000

British Library Cataloguing-in-Publication Data

A catalogue record for this book is available from the British Library

ISBN 0–85969–820–3

Typeset by Deltatype Limited, Birkenhead, Merseyside
Printed in Great Britain by
Biddles Ltd, Guildford and King's Lynn

Contents

For Emma, a delightful companion

Introduction: what Crohn's disease is and why it matters

Crohn's is essentially a disease of civilization – our own modern Western variety, and it is increasing alarmingly. By 1994 Professor Hermon-Taylor of St George's Hospital, London was calling it an epidemic. It used to be a rarity, and did not even have a name until the 1930s. It is still rare in the developing countries, although becoming less so as they 'catch' our lifestyle. It is particularly prevalent in the cities of North America, Western Europe and Australia. It is well known in New York, London, Sydney or Copenhagen, but not so common in sparsely populated rural areas such as Iceland and northern Norway.

How it was discovered

Although Crohn's disease acquired its name and identity only 70 years ago, as far back as 600 BC the Greek physician Asklepios was treating patients with bowel disorders. In his open-air health clinic they underwent a regimen of fasting, diet, rest and healing dreams (something like hypnosis). We would find this perfectly acceptable today. After the Greeks, hundreds of years went by – without any significant medical advances.

Much later, in 1769, Giovanni Morgagni described a young man with a chronic, debilitating illness with diarrhoea, which we might recognize today as Crohn's disease. At about the same time, Bonnie Prince Charlie complained of a persistent 'bloody flux' – this could have been the same problem. He cured himself by cutting out dairy products – a treatment still used today. In fact, in 1996 it was suggested by one group of doctors that mycobacteria in milk were the cause of the disease. In 1905, Dr Heinrich Albert Johne, in Germany, discovered a disease of the intestines in cattle that is very like Crohn's disease – but at that time no one had recognized the human version.

Dr Samuel Wilks of Guy's Hospital set the ball rolling in 1859 by writing and lecturing about his patient, Isabella Bankes, a recognizable – to us – Crohn's disease sufferer. Other colleagues became interested. In 1913, Dr Dalziel of Glasgow described a whole group of similar patients with what was still an illness without a name.

In 1930 Dr Burrill Crohn came on the scene. He was working at the Mount Sinai Hospital in New York, and at his wits' end over a 17-year-old patient. The boy had a high temperature, pain in the abdomen,

1

diarrhoea, and a tender lump in the appendix area. Dr Crohn suspected a tuberculous infection, but the youngster did not respond to the current treatment. A dangerous operation was the only way to find out what was wrong, but the situation became desperate and Dr Crohn's colleague, Dr A. A. Berg, decided to take the risk.

The lump turned out to be a hard mass of inflamed tissue at the lower end of the small intestine, the ileum. The big question was, what was causing the inflammation? Even today, although we have plenty of theories, we are still not sure. By 1932 Dr Crohn had searched out several more cases, and presented a paper about this 'new' illness at a meeting of the American Medical Association in New Orleans. He called it *regional ileitis* – inflammation of the ileum, usually the last part. (Classical or typical Crohn's disease is an inflammation of the ileum.) During the 1960s it became clear that the characteristic patches of inflammation, causing fever and diarrhoea, could crop up anywhere in the digestive tract, and the name *Crohn's disease* came to be used instead.

IBD

With the present day penchant for acronyms, IBD stands for *inflammatory bowel disease*, not to be confused with IBS, the common irritable bowel syndrome. IBD is an umbrella term doctors use for Crohn's disease and another illness called ulcerative colitis. The two illnesses are closely related, with similar, sometimes identical symptoms, but Crohn's is the more serious and more likely to be the forerunner of bowel cancer. Since the term IBD does not discriminate between the illnesses, the older name, Crohn's disease, is generally used.

Why does Crohn's disease matter so much?

- From Dr Crohn's time onwards, the illness has become increasingly prevalent, the numbers doubling between 1930 and 1970 and more than trebling since then.
- The key symptoms of pain and diarrhoea are unpleasant and socially embarrassing at best, exhausting and often disabling, and sometimes life-threatening at worst.
- New cases are appearing every day, in increasing numbers, and these tend to become chronic, with ups and down over the years.
- The most susceptible group is between ten and 40 years old, with a peak in the mid-twenties – years which are normally the most active and productive of your life, and among the happiest.

- While only three or four years ago it was almost unknown for Crohn's to start up in the under-tens or over-sixties, now this is happening more and more often.
- It tends to affect people in countries with a Western culture, but we do not know exactly where the risk lies, so that we can avoid it. We know it is not to do with social class or poverty. The one odd clue is that it is more likely to develop in people who were well-fed – not over-fed – as babies. A theory put forward in 1999 blaming the water supplies is not generally accepted.
- It can have a lasting damaging effect on development if it occurs in children. Youngsters with untreated Crohn's disease are liable to be short and sexually immature.
- There is no quick-fix cure, despite a range of treatment.
- Getting the best out of life when you have this illness means rejigging your whole lifestyle.

It applies to many illnesses, but to Crohn's especially: the sooner the problem is recognized and treatment begun the better the results, long term and short. This book explains the ways in which the disorder may show itself and the reasons behind the various treatments – including new, exciting research. Together we explore what you can do to get the very best out of life with Crohn's: the healthiest lifestyle and the various tricks and manoeuvres to beat this modern illness.

1

The digestive system: how it works

Imagine a life without eating and drinking – it would not be much fun. You would miss out on a recurrent pleasure, a comfort in distress and the centrepiece of your social life: from a formal banquet to a candle-lit supper for two, or fish and chips with the family. For happy eating you need a digestive system in good working order. It has to perform the everyday chemical magic of turning pizza and apple pie, or whatever you choose, into blood, brain and bone – all manufactured to your own individual specification.

To accomplish this miracle, the different parts of the digestive system have to co-ordinate their separate tasks. The timing is crucial: the food must pass down the alimentary tract (the pathway through the digestive system) at exactly the right rate for the processing to be completed of each of the varied ingredients of your meal – proteins, carbohydrates and fats. All of this would be pointless without the next stage: the absorption of the processed nutrients into the bloodstream, so that your body can use them. The main area for absorption is the small intestine, the part most seriously affected by Crohn's. The last task of the digestive system is the disposal of the waste matter – down the loo.

Crohn's disease upsets all this – absorption in particular, but also the basic work of digestion and elimination, and its timescale. To understand Crohn's it is a help to know the main parts of the digestive system, and what they do. Besides, it is a fascinating story.

The alimentary tract

The system operates under computer control. The computer is your brain, and it keeps in touch with every part through the nervous system. The two ends of the alimentary tract, the mouth and the anus, work in response to your conscious decisions – to eat and to go to the loo. All the rest comes under the influence of the autonomic (automatic) nervous system, and most of the activity is reflex, like a knee jerk. That is, given a particular stimulus, in this case tapping the front of your knee, your knee jerks automatically. You don't have to give it a thought.

Similarly, but in a much more complex way, the arrival of a fillet steak or a nut roast in your stomach stimulates a reflex reaction in the stomach glands. They produce just the right amount of pepsin to digest the type

4

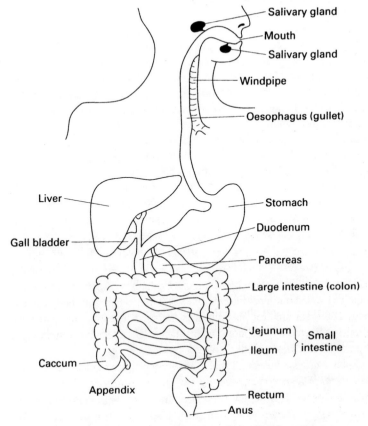

The alimentary tract: the pathway through the digestive system

and amount of protein. Imagine how tiresome it would be if you had to weigh and analyse what you ate, and then had to sit down with pencil and paper to work out which digestive enzymes you would need and the quantities. The whole system runs on a series of such reflexes.

Although Burrill Crohn in the 1930s believed Crohn's could affect only the last few inches of the ileum, the terminal part, by the 1960s other doctors had found that the tell-tale patches of inflammation could crop up anywhere in the alimentary tract. The effects – including your symptoms – differ according to the site of the trouble.

The mouth

This is the entry point for food, where tasting and savouring help you to decide whether to go ahead and enjoy or spit it out. One job of the mouth is to smash and crunch up the food: this allows the digestive juices to reach all parts of it and also makes it easier to swallow. The other important task depends on the salivary glands, the saliva factories: their output is about a litre per day. This slippery fluid lubricates each mouthful, making for easy transit down the oesophagus (gullet) to the stomach. It also contributes to oral hygiene by preventing crumbs of food sticking to the lining of the mouth, and washing away the germs which abound in the mouth.

Saliva has another useful role. It contains *ptyalin*, an enzyme which digests starch. You can test this out for yourself by chewing a piece of bread extra thoroughly. You will find it begins to taste sweet as the starch is digested into sugar. Gladstone had a point when he advised us to chew every mouthful 32 times, making a mush with the saliva well mixed in, and giving it time to work on the starch. An excellent start to digestion.

The salivary glands go into production when they receive information from the brain about the imminent arrival of food. My cat Emma dribbles in anticipation when she sees me open a tin of cat food. Our human reflexes are similar, and we speak of something delicious as 'mouth-watering'. The actual presence of food in the mouth also promotes a flow of saliva. Another stimulus to the flow of saliva is when the stomach has been irritated and you feel nauseous. The extra saliva helps to flush out the noxious material, or at least dilutes it.

The oesophagus

This flexible, collapsible tube connects the mouth with the stomach. It is lined, like the whole of the alimentary tract, by moist, delicate mucous membrane. Mucous glands down its length provide it with a protective covering. Food does not just fall down from the mouth to the stomach, but is massaged along by the muscles in the wall of the oesophagus. This is called *peristalsis*, and is a feature of the whole alimentary tract. It makes it possible for circus performers to drink a glass of water while standing on their heads. You can feel the peristalsis working if you accidentally swallow a plum stone or bolt a chunk of food without chewing it.

The 'law of the gut' is that throughout the alimentary tract, and most obviously in the oesophagus and the intestines, peristalsis moves the contents continuously onwards in the direction of the anus.

Lorna

Lorna had coped with her typical Crohn's quite effectively with the help of the standard drugs since she was 22. It was when she was 28 that some new symptoms appeared. Swallowing became uncomfortable, then increasingly difficult and she had an irritating cough. She lost three-quarters of a stone and looked ill. X-rays and passing an endoscope into her oesophagus showed Crohn's disease oesophagitis, with numerous small ulcers and a narrowing caused by a ring of swollen, inflamed tissue mixed with scarring. The treatment consisted of gently stretching this area by passing bougies (pencil-shaped instruments for pushing into narrow or blocked tubes) of increasing size through it. After five sessions Lorna was able to swallow normally again. Her medication was also adjusted and she was soon into a long period of remission.

The stomach

As food travels down the oesophagus the information is flashed forward to the stomach: 'Food on way'. The stomach muscles relax, especially at the entrance, and its glands begin to produce the digestive juices to deal with the type of foodstuff arriving.

The stomach has several important functions:

1 As a storage chamber for large quantities of food, so that you do not have to chomp all the time like a cow, but can take in all you need for the 24 hours at three or four meals.
2 Production of digestive juices, including hydrochloric acid to soften tough material, and *pepsin* to digest protein. This combination could be damaging to the body's own tissues, which is why there is a ring of muscle, the *pylorus*, that prevents the stomach contents running back into the oesophagus. The stomach lining is especially well coated with extra-strength mucus to protect it against the acid and pepsin, and in the duodenum, just past the exit from the stomach, the bile duct pours out its secretions. Bile is strongly alkaline and neutralizes the acid.
  The stomach enzymes can digest carbohydrates as well as proteins.
3 Production of *intrinsic factor*, another constituent of the stomach juices. This is necessary for the absorption of vitamin B12, without which a serious form of anaemia develops: pernicious anaemia.
4 Kneading and thoroughly mixing the food and the stomach juices, for as long as it takes, to produce a milky-looking semi-fluid called *chyme*.
5 Slow, controlled emptying of the chyme into the small intestine, as and when facilities for the next stage become available. There must obviously be room, and the rate of emptying is geared to allow for the digestive process to continue until the chyme is ready for absorption.

The correct rate of transit is of key importance to the digestive process, and nervous messages are sent both ways between the stomach and the small intestine, for instance, information that the chyme is still too acid, or contains too much undigested fat or protein – or is irritating for some other reason.

6 Stomach reflexes: the automatic message from the stomach to the small intestine is called the *gastroenteric reflex*, while the reverse, the *enterogastric reflex*, tells the stomach to turn off the production of acid and pepsin, because the chyme has moved on into the intestine. (Any strong emotion has an equally powerful switch-off effect on the stomach.) Messages from the stomach to the colon set off the *gastrocolic reflex*. This alerts the colon to the arrival into the system of another meal, and this is often a good time to get rid of accumulated waste matter as, for instance, the after-breakfast bowel movement.

The small intestine

This comprises, in order, the duodenum, the jejunum and the ileum. Its smallness refers to the relative narrowness of the tube compared with the much wider colon or large intestine, but it is many times longer. The gastroenteric reflex stimulates increased peristalsis in the small intestine, especially the jejunum, the first part after the duodenum. The normal travel time from the stomach to the caecum, where the large intestine begins, is between three and five hours, depending on the type and quantity of food in the system.

The *duodenum* is only a few inches long, little more than a lobby to the stomach. Partly because it is more exposed to the stomach juices than the lower parts of the intestine, ulcers often develop here. The most important role of the duodenum is the reception, through the bile duct, of digestive juices from the pancreas, and bile made by the liver and stored in the gall bladder. The pancreatic enzymes are geared for the digestion of all three kinds of foodstuff – proteins, fats and carbohydrates. Bile is essential for the digestion and preparation for absorption of fats, a necessary requirement for a body to obtain its supplies of the fat-soluble vitamins A, D, E and K. The gall bladder automatically pours out all the bile it is storing when a fatty meal arrives in the duodenum.

The *jejunum* and *ileum* comprise the rest of the small intestine, coils many feet long. In the first part, the jejunum, peristalsis is vigorous and also other muscular movements which ensure that the chyme is thoroughly mixed with the digestive juices, making a runny mish-mash. The digestive process continues as the chyme travels through the jejunum and is virtually complete when it reaches the ileum, the organ most affected by Crohn's. The ileum has the important task of absorbing almost all the nutrients from the chyme into the bloodstream, a role for which it is specifically adapted.

Its lining is covered with tiny, delicate fingers of tissue which both release liquid and reabsorb it when it is loaded with nourishment from the chyme. Another special feature of the cells lining the small intestine is their short life – five to seven days. The advantage of this is that any damage is quickly repaired with brand new cells, indicating how indispensable the ileum is to life. If there is some irritation in the small intestine, such as inflammation or the presence of bacteria, the movement of the chyme is speeded up, resulting in copious, watery diarrhoea. This washes out germs or other irritants, but also causes the loss of essential nourishment.

Every day, when you are in normal health, your ileum absorbs into the bloodstream:

- several hundred grams of carbohydrate· (100 g is equivalent to $3\frac{1}{2}$ ounces, or nearly a quarter of a pound)
- 100 g of fat
- 50–100 g of protein constituents (amino acids)
- 50–100 g of chemical ions, such as iron, calcium and magnesium
- all the vitamins (naturally-occurring compounds needed in small quantities for normal metabolism and bodily function, but which the human body cannot make for itself)
- 7–8 litres of fluid (a litre is the equivalent of about two pints)

The ileum is capable of absorbing much larger quantities if necessary: up to 20 litres of water in a day, for instance. Although the ileum is the main area for absorption, other parts of the digestive system can take in some substances. The stomach, for example, can absorb alcohol – the reason for its rapid effect – and several drugs, such as aspirin, and the duodenum absorbs calcium, so long as there is also some vitamin D available. The colon can only absorb water, and a few simple chemicals dissolved in it.

The large intestine

The ileum ends in the *ileocaecal junction*, where there is a double ring of muscles to regulate when and at what rate the now depleted chyme is allowed through. It is reduced to about $1\frac{1}{2}$ litres (1500 ml) daily. The caecum is a bulge that marks the beginning of the large intestine. It is in the lower right-hand corner of the abdomen and the appendix is a short blind alley which comes off it. The caecum continues as the colon until it becomes the specialized end section, the rectum, and the final exit, the anus.

The first half of the colon is called the 'absorbing colon' since it absorbs most of the water and chemicals entering it, leaving about 100 ml for the waste mixture: the motions or faeces. The second part is the 'storage colon' where the waste is kept until there is a signal that it is time to empty it. There are normally many bacteria in the colon, especially 'colon bacilli', and they are responsible for the gas or flatus that can be so embarrassing, produced from various foods such as beans, cabbage and unabsorbable roughage.

The only material produced in the colon is mucus, and its lining is massed with mucus cells. These are stimulated by the presence of waste matter, and the mucus protects and lubricates the lining. It also helps to bind the waste – or faecal – matter together, for convenience in storage and disposal. The contents of the colon are semi-liquid at the caecal end, mushy in the middle and semi-solid when they reach the rectum.

When the colon is irritated by inflammation, enteritis or inadequately digested material, it reacts by pouring out more mucus and speeding up the passage of its contents by mass movements involving its whole length. Emotional disturbances stimulate the colon to produce a large amount of ropey mucus, which produces the urge to pass a motion as often as every half-hour – although there are no faeces to pass.

Andrew

Andrew was a conscientious 18-year-old, predictably screwed up about his A-level examination. He had 'always' had a tendency to diarrhoea when he was upset, as a child, so no one took much notice this time. However, after one sharp attack the symptoms kept recurring, and he noticed what he called 'muck' in his motions. This consisted of bloodstained mucus and pus. Andrew had Crohn's disease affecting his colon: Crohn's colitis. It responded well to a drug called sulphasalazine, an old favourite in Crohn's.

The *rectum* and *anus* comprise the final parts of the alimentary tract and differ from the previous sections in that you have some conscious control over them. The sensitive rectum informs you when it is full and reminds you to go to the loo. The muscle of the anus has to relax to allow the motion to pass, and this is under your control so that you can wait for a convenient time and place. The anal region is especially sensitive, and inflammation here, *proctitis*, can be so painful that the victim is afraid to let the motions through.

The motion

A normal motion consists of 75 per cent water and 25 per cent solids; these in turn include 30 per cent dead bacteria and their products, 30 per cent indigestible fibre, and 10 to 20 per cent fat. Too much water means diarrhoea and too little leads to constipation, while excess of fat gives a bulky, pale putty-coloured stool. Blood, pus or mucus in the motion are all abnormal.

The emotional input

No one would suggest that Crohn's and its serious symptoms are 'all in the mind', but it would be unrealistic to claim that your feelings have no part to play in the working of your digestive system. It stands to reason that you cannot feel happy when you have stomach pain or diarrhoea, but it is also true that emotional stress can bring on physical symptoms, or make them worse.

Long before Sigmund Freud, in 1895, blamed bowel disorders on emotional conflict, or psychosomatics became fashionable in the 1950s, it was taken for granted that there was an intimate link between feelings and the bowels. In the Bible, Solomon, referring to a friend, said, 'My bowels were moved for him', and St John wrote of 'the bowels of compassion'. In the seventeenth century John Gay's Macheath appealed to Lucy: 'Have you no bowels, no tenderness?', while more crudely, today, we connect the bowels with courage. If we say that someone 'hasn't got the guts for it', we are talking not anatomy but feelings.

Physicians and surgeons both focus on the physical aspects of Crohn's disease and argue over the relative merits of medicine and surgery in this illness. You, the sufferer, are in no position to join the argument on scientific grounds. Where you do have the edge is in the vast area of mind and emotions. Only you know your feelings, your hopes and your fears and what you find stressful in your life. They cannot be analysed chemically, X-rayed or measured in millilitres, yet this part of you is involved in everything that happens in your body. The connection is obvious when you think of what happens when you are frightened or anxious. Your heart speeds up, your saliva dries up, and sometimes your bowels 'turn to water'.

You cannot switch on a calm, confident mood when you are feeling distressed, any more than you can will away a pain in your stomach or diarrhoea. The psychological and emotional aspects of Crohn's require consideration as well as the physical side.

Never forget that you are a whole person.

2

Are you at risk? The background to Crohn's disease

Most people do not develop Crohn's disease, and you do not want to be one of the unlucky ones. What are the risks and is there anything you can do to lessen them? Unfortunately it is not as simple in Crohn's as it is, for instance, with measles. In that case we know what causes it – the measles virus – and can alert our immunity system, or our children's, by vaccination. We have not pinpointed the cause of Crohn's, but are fairly sure that it is a mix of several factors – none of which we know for certain. There are a few pointers, but no definite answers, despite the best endeavours of research workers over the last 70 years.

Epidemiology – the numbers game – can tell us how many people in different places and different circumstances develop the disease. This body count, since it affects whole communities, not just individuals, provides some clues as to risk. It shows up the influence of race and family – the genetic input – compared with environmental factors such as lifestyle, stress and diet.

The recent huge increase in the number of cases in the West must be to do with lifestyle rather than genetics – you cannot change your parents or your ancestry, but how and where you live can certainly alter. Your job, or your partner's, can take you to New York or New Delhi, or you may choose to move from town to country or vice versa – or go vegetarian.

There must be something (or probably several items) in our so-called civilized Western way of life which makes us more susceptible to Crohn's than, for example, Zimbabweans or Nicaraguans. Whatever it is, it is getting worse. The importance of lifestyle on a country-wide basis is borne out by the increasing prevalence of Crohn's in the Western world, and its even more dramatic upsurge in developing countries which are currently Westernizing, with industry replacing agriculture and a shift of population to the towns. This has been well documented in New Zealand, South Africa and in the black population of America.

Town or country

In Wales, Scotland, Northern Ireland, Portugal and Galicia, where statistics have been collected, proportionately more cases of Crohn's are found in the towns, especially where there is much industry, than in rural

12

areas. This applies all over Europe. The instinct to retire to the country is a healthy one, but it comes too late to lessen the risk of Crohn's since the peak age for developing it is 26.

Diet

No one type of diet, whether Mediterranean, Indian, vegetarian, plain English or sophisticated French, is particularly associated with more or less Crohn's disease. But there are a few significant dietary pointers.

Sugar

It has been shown recently that people with Crohn's disease habitually eat much more sugar than the average – 150 per cent more in Birmingham, 120 per cent more in Tel-Aviv, 110 per cent more in Dusseldorf, and 40 per cent more in Manchester. It is not certain whether the excess sugar makes Crohn's more likely, or if Crohn's itself gives you a sweet tooth.

Fruit and vegetables

Statistically, Crohn's disease sufferers eat far less fruit and vegetables than other people. Twenty-five per cent have one portion or less of these foods daily, and hardly any hit the UK recommended guideline of five portions plus per day. This is likely to have been a long-term pattern, present before Crohn's as well as after.

Fillers

Because of their small intake of green and yellow vegetables and fruit, those who develop Crohn's are often heavy users of filler foods. They eat more potatoes, pasta, bread, biscuits, cake and breakfast cereals than the rest of us. At one time cornflakes came under the spotlight, but since they are usually eaten with milk and sugar, both suspect, it was impossible to come to a firm conclusion about whether they were truly a risk factor.

Sometimes a whole extended family may go for the same old favourites: bangers and mash, cornflakes, crisps, chips and biscuits – with most things well sugared. Such families are more likely than others to have members suffering from Crohn's and ulcerative colitis.

Processed foods

Crohn's disease patients tend to go for these convenience foods more than most. Can there, after all, be something harmful in additives, preservatives and flavour-enhancers? Some people have a vague idea that in Crohn's the body is reacting to some mysterious, unidentified ingredient in our food – perhaps to do with processing?

Poultry

Oddly, the only meats that seem relevant are the ubiquitous chicken and turkey. These have become increasingly popular since red meat has had such a bad press, and Crohn's patients eat more poultry than the rest of us. Much of it is bought in supermarkets, processed and packaged.

Milk

Groups of researchers, over the years, have suspected dairy products of being one of the roots of the trouble. In a study of American veterans with Crohn's there were many more who stayed in remission (not permanently cured, but without symptoms pro tem) among a section who were not allowed dairy products, compared with those on full service rations. (And then there was Bonnie Prince Charlie.) In only the last five years there has been a serious suggestion that milk contaminated with mycobacterium paratuberculosis is a prime cause of Crohn's. There is also the matter of lactase deficiency (see p. 94). However, for many patients, disappointingly, cutting out this valuable nourishment seems to make no difference.

Caffeine

The habit of using an excess of this universal stimulant, in coffee, tea and cola drinks, also slightly increases the risk of Crohn's disease.

Food intolerance

This may underlie Crohn's in some cases (see p. 93). The evidence is indirect and comprises miraculous improvement for some people if a particular item of food is removed from their diet. It is not that Crohn's is an allergic reaction, since it takes quite large quantities of food to bring on the symptoms. In fact a trial lasting seven days is now standard for testing for food intolerance. The food being tested is disguised in a blackcurrant drink or lentil soup – or even delivered straight into the stomach through a tube – so there is no preconceived bias. A positive reaction is the appearance of Crohn's symptoms: pain and diarrhoea. A wide range of foods has been implicated. The figures in the brackets in the list below are percentages of Crohn's patients who reacted positively in a food test.

- wheat (28)
- dairy products (24)

- brassicas, cabbage family (16)
- maize, corn (12)
- yeast (11)
- tomatoes (11)
- citrus fruits (10)
- eggs (10)
- tapwater, coffee, bananas, potatoes, lamb (8)
- pork (7)
- beef, rice (5)
- tea (4)
- fish (3)
- onions (2)
- chicken, barley, rye, turkey, alcohol, chocolate, shellfish, swede and additives (1)

The patient is put on an elemental diet (see p. 96) and different foods are reintroduced one by one, stopping the process if there is pain or diarrhoea. Patients who respond favourably to diet changes are still well two years later, in two-thirds of cases.

There is a theory that it is not the particular food in itself that sets off Crohn's disease, but its effect on the bacteria that normally inhabit the gut.

Philip

Philip was small, in particular he was short for his age, 12, when he developed Crohn's disease. His mother had a full-time job and he was an only child. He was an independent youngster and took a pride in managing for himself when his mother was at work. He could have chosen a snack of bread and cheese and helped himself from the fruit dish when he was hungry, but what he went for were crisps, chocolate bars, and sometimes a bowl of Frosties – sugar-dipped cornflakes. Even at weekends, when his mother cooked the standard meat and two vegetables, Philip preferred ham from a packet with chips, followed by a gooey sweet. His choice of food did nothing to hinder the development of Crohn's. However, diet alone could not have been responsible for the illness: there must also have been other genetic or environmental factors at work.

Smoking

It has been found that the proportion of smokers among Crohn's sufferers is higher than average. This applies to their current smoking habit and also what it was before the illness came on. The link with tobacco is stronger in the towns and cities of the UK than, for instance, in Chicago or Denver. The risk is cumulative, so the more heavily you smoke or the longer the period when you have been a smoker, the greater the risk. For an average smoker there is four times the normal risk. It is not only the risk of developing the disease in the first place; the chances of recurrence are also increased, and it is likely to be more serious. The likelihood of needing an operation is greater for Crohn's patients who continue with their smoking.

The contraceptive pill

This too, poses an increased risk of Crohn's disease, particularly if a high oestrogen preparation is used. Back in 1968, when the Pill was still under close scrutiny, it was discovered that, like smoking, the Pill was associated in some mysterious way with damage to the tiny blood vessels in the lining of the colon. There was an increased risk of Crohn's, especially of the colon rather than the ileum.

In one review, 75 per cent of women aged 40 or less who had Crohn's were on the Pill, compared with 31 per cent of other women of the same age. The risk of Crohn's is doubled for those on the Pill, and if they have taken it for more than five years the risk is up to eight times the norm. On the other hand, if they come off it the extra risk declines to nothing over five years.

HRT (hormone replacement therapy)

Since this contains the same hormones as the Pill, it seems likely that it carries the same risks, but there are fewer cases of Crohn's disease in the middle-aged than the young, so they figure less in research studies.

Constipation

Long-term constipation, with the non-stop use of laxatives, is considered by some to predispose to both IBD and irritable bowel syndrome. It is so common that any effect must be minute.

Kirsty
Kirsty liked to live life to the full. She had started smoking at 13, alcohol about the same time, and she went on the Pill almost as soon as her periods were established. She had a lot of boyfriends, then men friends, and after a couple of marriages ending in divorce she was still

only 35, and enjoying a child-free sex life. Her career prospered as a secretary turned administrator; and then she lost her appetite and dropped half a stone without trying. She felt tired – unusual for her – and the GP, who knew she had a cousin with ulcerative colitis, referred her to a specialist. He diagnosed IBD but did not subject her to unpleasant invasive investigations to see whether it was Crohn's or ulcerative colitis causing her symptoms. If they settled down there would be no definitive sign of either illness anyway. The GP had, of course, known that having a relative with ulcerative colitis increased Kirsty's likelihood of developing either form of IBD.

Kirsty had several months of treatment with a battery of drugs. She came off the Pill and the cigarettes, and with her positive spirit, rebuilt her life. She has also remarried and plans to have a family.

Micro-organisms (germs)

Back in 1913, Dr Kennedy Dalziel found that there was a similar illness to Crohn's disease – an illness as yet without a name – in cows, due to a mycobacterium very like, but not the same as, that which causes tuberculosis of the intestines in humans.

Seventeen years later, Dr Crohn and his colleagues continued the hunt for a mycobacterium in the tissues of their Crohn's disease patients. Like a relay race, others took up the challenge, and in 1978 they struck oil. A group of four researchers found mycobacterium paratuberculosis in the tissues of one single patient with Crohn's. (*Para* means *like*, as in paramedic.) In 1984, the microbe was found in four more patients, then in some macaque monkeys. The stumbling block that meant the research took so many years was the inordinate length of time – up to eight months – that it took for the mycobacterium to grow in culture. The earlier workers must often have given up hope of any bacteria developing. Now we have the recipe for a culture medium which this pernickety bug really likes: veal broth with yeast extract, horse serum, sugar and a few other choice ingredients.

Mycobacterium paratuberculosis and one of its close relatives are found in as many as a third of Crohn's patients. This must mean that it is implicated in some way. Further evidence of mycobacterial involvement is the occasional dramatic improvement in the patient's symptoms using antimycobacterial antibiotics such as streptomycin, and in the last two years lesser known drugs such a rifabutin. The big problem is the lack of consistency. Viruses have also been investigated, and some unusual organisms, such as Pseudomonas, have come under suspicion, but studies have been disappointingly inconclusive.

Another germ theory is that in Crohn's there is a fault in the lining of the gut, which allows bacteria that normally cause no trouble to penetrate the surface and produce the patches of inflammation that comprise Crohn's. Suspect bugs include *Streptococcus faecalis* and *E. (Escherichia) coli* and of course, *Mycobacterium paratuberculosis*. The weakness of the lining membrane would be something you are born with, from your genes.

Rather than any particular micro-organism causing Crohn's directly, it is more likely that it predisposes the person to the illness, but this only breaks out when there are other influences at work – faults in the gut lining or in the immune system, or some of the adverse dietary and lifestyle factors. A large number of people may, for instance, be harbouring the mycobacterium, but only a few develop the symptoms. Some people may be hypersensitive to the particular microbe, or their immune system has in some way been primed to react in the wrong way.

A natural phenomenon that can confuse the issue is that different causes may produce the same effect on the body. For example, we all know that a headache may be the result of alcohol or another drug, a migraine, sinus infection, a stuffy room – or anxiety. In Crohn's there may need to be more than one adverse factor or several acting together to produce the disorder.

Defects in the immune system

Another current notion proposes that Crohn's disease is an abnormal reaction by the immune system, either to something that is normally harmless, or perhaps to a toxin left behind by a germ that has passed through the body. All this is speculative, but a great deal of work is in progress. It is a fingers crossed situation.

Steroid medicines

To add to the confusion, while steroid medicines often suppress Crohn's disease symptoms in the short term, if they are used continuously their long-term effects actually reduce the chances of remission. (This is in contrast to the wholly beneficial effect of steroids in ulcerative colitis, the other IBD.)

Your genes

Important though environmental factors are, the genetic input through your family connections has an enormous individual effect. If you have a brother or sister with Crohn's, you run 30 times the risk of developing the illness compared with the general population – and a staggering 67 times if you are identical twins. The risk is only about 13 times the norm if you have a parent or other first-degree relative with the illness: equally this applies to any child you may have. One curious fact is that if you suffer from Crohn's you are more likely to have relatives with ulcerative colitis than with Crohn's itself.

These risks may sound alarming, but to get them in perspective remember that the chances of developing Crohn's for the general population are small – say 16 out of 100,000 people per year. Even multiplied by 30, this does not amount to many. Of course there are more Crohn's cases in the most vulnerable age group, those in their mid-twenties, but even among these the numbers are still relatively small. In 1996 among all those aged 26 in the UK, the proportion diagnosed as having Crohn's came out at 30 per 10,000.

Sex, which is a genetic factor, makes no difference to your likelihood of getting Crohn's, apart from one small, fairly rare group where sex is indirectly involved. In these cases the gene passes from mother to son only, the so-called X-linked inheritance. The illness always starts up in childhood, and often affects a large part of the small intestine.

A more dramatic genetic link affects the whole Jewish race, particularly the Ashkenazi line. They run between eight and thirteen times the normal risk of Crohn's disease, no matter where they live – London, New York, Tel-Aviv or Paris. This seems to be based on a metabolic quirk, also genetic. They tend to have a shortage of *lactase*, an enzyme which is used in the digestion of milk. Although this suggests that milk products should be avoided, by Jewish people especially, it is only one factor among many and may have an insignificant effect by itself. Of the 'Western' countries, Israel has the greatest proportion of Crohn's sufferers, partly due to the genetic effect, but also because it is still actively developing industrially.

Rachel

Rachel's grandparents had left Germany in 1939, in the nick of time, and by a circuitous route reached Australia. Rachel was a good, third-generation Aussie, fit and sporty. In fact she excelled at swimming and was a junior champion at one time. Naturally she had a healthy lifestyle – no cigarettes, plenty of fruit and vegetables, moderate alcohol and regular exercise – so it came as a shock when she developed Crohn's disease. There had been some question of an uncle of hers having a serious bowel problem, but he was in Europe and not in close touch. There was also a distant cousin who was prone to bouts of diarrhoea, but she had been put down as 'neurotic'. There was no doubt about the seriousness of Rachel's illness, however, and she had to have an urgent operation. Her basically excellent health stood her in good stead in this crisis, and she made a smooth recovery from her surgery which had successfully removed the affected part of her small intestine. She is now back in training – after several months concentrating on her recovery.

Psychological and emotional risk factors

It cannot be doubted that there is an interplay between psychological events and physical symptoms, but for Crohn's disease it is not a simple matter of cause and effect. Some personality types and some less permanent emotional states, such as depression or anxiety, may predispose you to Crohn's, and some stressful events may precipitate an attack, particularly when you already have the illness but it is quiescent.

Psychological shocks and strains may act as triggers, for example, bereavement, divorce, being burgled or getting into debt, a new job or its opposite, becoming redundant. Physical stresses with emotional tie-ups include a severe infection, pregnancy, your first period. Even the good news events, like getting married or winning the lottery, act as a stress, and if you are a Crohn's sufferer your bowels are your weak spot.

People who develop Crohn's disease are usually stable, conscientious and reliable; they are not given to exaggeration or complaining unnecessarily. In fact, although they are sensitive, they tend to hide their hurt. Like anyone else, if you fall into a depression or an anxiety state, you are more vulnerable to illness, and this includes Crohn's. Equally, it is lowering to your spirits when you are going through an attack of the disease, and of course you feel anxious about the outcome.

The psychological aspects of Crohn's are touched upon in Chapters 1 and 9, but are dealt with more fully in Chapter 11.

Leonard

Leonard was a teacher at a primary school. At 24 he had been teaching for only a year when the abdominal pains began. He tried to ignore them. He had always wanted to teach and share the pleasure he derived from his chosen subject, history. He found his life at the school was a roller-coaster of delights and disasters, with the emphasis on the latter. Despite the niggling pain, he managed to cope with the day-to-day hurdles until he succumbed to a nasty bout of 'flu. It was when he was recovering from that that the bowel symptoms came out in full force. The depression that commonly follows influenza merged with his depression over his Crohn's disease. Both required treatment.

The causes of Crohn's are *multifactorial* – that is, there must be a concurrence of several different factors, genetic and environmental, acting together to enable the disease to develop. In the light of Professor Hermon-Taylor's theories, even drinking tap water may pose a risk – for the very vulnerable (see p. 129).

3

Signs and symptoms: how Crohn's disease shows itself

Crohn's disease, although not a killer, is troublesome enough to interfere with your life disastrously – if you let it. So the sooner the illness is diagnosed and treatment is started the better: you suffer less and learn to adapt to the lifestyle that suits you best. The first step is down to you. If you notice anything unusual or uncomfortable about your bowels or your abdomen, and it does not settle down in a few days, and especially if you have any of the symptoms listed below, do not bravely ignore them. Have them checked out. It will probably turn out to be nothing of importance, but it is worthwhile to be sure.

Crohn's can first appear in several different guises. Usually it comes on insidiously, creeping up almost imperceptibly at first, and either getting gradually but steadily worse or manifesting in little bouts of symptoms which become increasingly frequent. Less often there is a sudden, explosive start to the illness, with dramatic symptoms of pain, vomiting and diarrhoea.

Common symptoms

The big three are: pain, diarrhoea and undernutrition.

The key symptoms may not be the first warning. Look out for any of these:

Pain in the abdomen

In Crohn's this is likely to be in the lower right hand corner, the appendix area. Most frequently it is constant rather than throbbing or colicky. Often you can notice a slight fulness, not quite a bulge, in the area, and it may be tender to pressure. This is due to the pain and swelling of inflamed tissues, particularly the peritoneum, the sensitive membrane which covers the intestines.

If there is a degree of obstruction, causing a build-up of its contents, the intestine wall is stretched, and registers this as pain. Slight, partial obstruction may be due to the inflamed lining itself, a band of tough, fibrous scar tissue, or muscle spasm. In the colon and rectum such spasms are called *colorectal cramps*. There can also be muscle spasms in the small intestine, or that other part of the alimentary tube, the oesophagus. Muscle spasms may be set off by inflammation or the irritation of incompletely digested food arriving in the affected part, but typically they are a symptom of the muscle pushing hard to get material past a narrow or more seriously blocked section of the gut. In this situation the pain is colicky, and you feel it in the centre of your abdomen.

'Tummy rumbles'

These may be loud and excessive if your intestinal muscles are having to work extra hard to keep things moving. Their posh name is *borborygmi*.

Poor appetite (anorexia)

Everything may taste different, or seem to have no taste or smell, or at any rate not an appetizing one; and you feel full after only a few mouthfuls. There is no pleasure in eating.

Nausea

If this develops you will not want to eat at all. Anorexia, nausea and sometimes diarrhoea may all be due to a lack of vitamins or trace minerals like zinc: a vicious circle if you are not eating properly. A more likely cause for nausea, however, is a direct effect of Crohn's on your stomach and duodenum. In 8 per cent of people with Crohn's there are visible signs of the trouble if the doctor looks into the stomach with a flexible fibreoptic telescope: an endoscope. In 24 per cent there is an abnormal X-ray.

In Crohn's disease the stomach passes the food into the small intestine more slowly than normally. This is due to the 'ileal brake'. The ileum is almost always affected and cannot absorb the nourishment in your food effectively. This means that the material that the ileum passes on is not fully digested and it irritates the colon at the ileocaecal junction. The ring of muscle there clamps down to slow down, if not completely prevent, the flow of irritating stuff. This slow-down or 'brake' produces a back pressure all the way back to the stomach. The whole system of appetite, eating and being nourished is upset, a measure of how important an illness this is.

Vomiting

This may be a symptom of obstruction of the gut, or part of an acute phase, when the whole digestive system is in turmoil.

Lump in the abdomen

Sometimes you – or the doctor – can feel a definite lump in the painful part of your abdomen. This is made up of coils of small intestine stuck together by the inflammatory process. It is not a cancer, and not serious in itself.

Raised temperature

This goes with any inflammation, but is likely to be slight in Crohn's, unless it arises in the type which comes on acutely. The average normal temperature is between 36.7 and 37°C, or 98 to 98.6°F.

Malaise

This comprises a vague feeling of being under par, or 'having an off day' – which goes on and on. Even if there's nothing definitely wrong, you just do not feel right.

Diarrhoea

This means frequent motions. They may be loose and semi-liquid or fully-formed, bulky and pale, but the daily quantity is well above normal. Diarrhoea may originate in either the small or the large intestine. A large volume of liquid, passed with more inconvenience than pain, suggests that the ileum is to blame. If there is pain, with blood, pus and mucus in the motion, the colon is directly involved. There may be an uncomfortable feeling in the rectum all the time, and sometimes there is a strong urge to pass a motion with only a little mucus to show for it (tenesmus).

Other abdominal symptoms

You may have any of these:

- Bloating, so that your abdomen seems enormous except first thing in the morning.
- Excessive flatus, so that you keep wanting to fart.
- Dyspepsia – discomfort after meals.
- Heartburn.

Undernutrition

This means a lack of essential nourishment. It arises in Crohn's for three main reasons:

- Eating too little because of poor appetite.
- Losing nourishment through diarrhoea and vomiting.
- Failure of the small intestine to absorb properly not only the bulk of the major nutrients, carbohydrates, fats and proteins but the equally essential vitamins and minerals, even though only tiny amounts of these are necessary. If your ileum is ill and unable to work normally – the situation in Crohn's – it does not matter how well-balanced your diet is, you cannot get the goodness from it.

Shortness of stature

This is noticeable in those whose Crohn's had begun to develop before or during their adolescent growth spurt. Sometimes the illness starts, quietly, long before the tell-tale symptoms appear.

Eileen

Eileen was a 20-year-old student who found she kept getting a pain in the right side of her abdomen. One day it was worse than usual and she felt 'ropey' so she took her temperature and found that it was slightly raised at 37.5°C (99.7°F). She decided to consult the college doctor. He found Eileen's appendix area was tender and he also detected some guarding, a protective tightening of the muscles over the place which was hurting. Eileen felt sick but she did not vomit. The doctor sent her off to hospital with a provisional diagnosis of acute appendicitis.

At the hospital a blood test showed an excess of white cells (leucocytosis) such as occurs in appendicitis and other inflammatory conditions. The commonplace operation of appendicectomy seemed the obvious thing to do. In the event the surgeon found that Eileen's appendix was perfectly healthy, but the last few inches of her ileum were swollen and sore. The inflammation was well established, healing in some parts while spreading in others, so it must have been developing over several months – without her realizing anything was amiss. The surgeon took a tiny sample of the affected tissue, and it confirmed what he had suspected – that Eileen had Crohn's disease. The operation did no harm, but uncovered the real diagnosis. Treatment was started forthwith, in this case with sulphasalazine, a well-tried stand-by in Crohn's.

Debbie

Debbie was in sales. She was 38 and had always been slim, but recently she had had several bouts of diarrhoea and lost a few pounds. That was why it was so distressing to find her abdomen blowing up whenever she had a meal, so that it bulged out – 'as though I was pregnant', she complained. The GP tried various ploys but they did not help, and he finally sent Debbie to a female gastroenterologist (Debbie was an ardent feminist). The specialist arranged a special type of X-ray involving a barium infusion (see p. 50) which showed ulcers in the lining of the ileum and a narrowing (stenosis) in one part. These were the clues to the diagnosis of Crohn's disease.

The first medication Debbie was given was a steroid, which settled

25

her abdomen quickly, and this was followed by azathioprine, a better treatment in the long term.

Malabsorption

The principal feature of Crohn's disease is damage to the small intestine, so that it cannot do its job of absorbing the nourishment from your food. This is malabsorption.

Effects of malabsorption:

- Loss of weight in adults.
- Slow-down of growth and development in children, particularly growth in height and sexual development.
- Loss of protein: this sets off a vicious circle of diarrhoea and increased loss of weight, with muscle weakness and wasting; there may also be swelling of the ankles and hands, and sometimes the face.
- Passing of undigested fat in the motions, involving loss of the fat-soluble vitamins, A and D.
- Inadequate absorption of carbohydrates, the major fillers in your diet, and the usual fuel for running your brain and all your body processes. Milk sugar, lactose, is particularly poorly absorbed because of a deficiency in the necessary enzyme. Some Crohn's sufferers are intolerant to milk products and react to them with colic, bloating, wind and sometimes diarrhoea.

Vitamin and mineral deficiencies

Vitamin A (retinol)

A lack can cause dry, uncomfortable eyes and 'night blindness' – poor vision in twilight condition. It has been called the anti-infection vitamin, because it helps to protect the mucous membranes, for instance in your throat and the alimentary tract, from infection.

Vitamin D (calciferol)

A shortage produces an inability to absorb and use calcium, which is necessary for the health and strength of bones and teeth.

Vitamin B12 (cobalamin)

It is needed for the formation of red blood corpuscles. A lack leads to a serious form of anaemia, pernicious anaemia, with weakness and tiredness, pale skin, sore tongue and bouts of diarrhoea. The nervous system, including the brain, may be affected.

Folate

This acts in conjunction with vitamin B12. A lack of either increases the effects of a lack of the other.

Iron

A deficiency leads to simple anaemia, with such symptoms as fatigue, dizziness, shortness of breath, palpitations, headache, dim vision and swollen ankles – but often these symptoms are slight and are ignored.

Magnesium

This is required by the nerves which service the muscles. A lack leads to a tremor and odd, involuntary muscular movements, and sometimes depression or a muddled feeling. It has a key role in the metabolism of sugars and starches.

Calcium

A shortage in adults leads to osteoporosis, and in children to weak, faulty bones (rickets) and poor teeth.

Zinc

A deficiency can cause diarrhoea, eczema round the mouth and general apathy. In children growth and sexual development in particular are held back.

For practical purposes, if you have any vague symptoms of tiredness or muscle weakness and you have been losing weight over a matter of weeks, it is worthwhile discussing with your doctor whether you should have a check for deficiency of any of these vitamins and minerals.

When the colon is affected

Often both the small intestine and the colon (large intestine) are involved in Crohn's disease, and in a minority the colon only is affected – Crohn's colitis. Crohn's colitis is almost indistinguishable from ulcerative colitis, the other IBD.

The symptoms are:

- Diarrhoea is the key symptom, with blood, pus and mucus in the motions. Blood is particularly likely in the over-forties. In the occasional case there is constipation instead of diarrhoea.
- Fast heart rate (tachycardia): you can feel it in your chest and count it

by your pulse. More than 90 beats a minute is abnormally fast unless you are exercising.

- High, swinging temperature, at its highest in the evening.
- Swollen, tender abdomen.
- Tenesmus – you feel you want to pass a motion even when there is nothing there.
- Oedema – swelling due to water-logging of the tissues, affecting your ankles and hands. If you press your finger into the swollen part it leaves a little pit which takes a few seconds to go back to normal.
- Tags of swollen (oedematous) skin round the anus.

The colitis type of Crohn's usually comes on as an acute attack with the symptoms at their worst. It may be mistaken for food-poisoning – gastroenteritis – initially, but in the case of Crohn's there is a tendency for the illness to persist and become chronic. The acute symptoms die down but do not disappear completely. Every now and then there is an acute exacerbation, but these recurrences are hardly ever as severe as the first attack.

Daniel

Daniel, 50, thought he 'had eaten something' when he was suddenly seized with diarrhoea streaked with blood and his whole abdomen felt sore and tender. His temperature was nearly 40°C. His doctor also thought gastroenteritis was the likeliest cause but took a stool sample and reassured Daniel that he expected the symptoms to settle down within 48 to 72 hours. They did not, and the stool sample did not contain salmonella or any of the other common culprits. The GP then referred Daniel to the nearest major hospital, where a colonoscopy (fibreoptic examination of the colon) was carried out. It showed the 'cobblestone' appearance of the lining of the colon, characteristic of Crohn's disease. After an initial course of steroids, Daniel did well on loperamide.

Illnesses which may be mistaken for Crohn's disease

- Gastroenteritis or food-poisoning, as in Daniel's case.
- Ulcerative colitis: sometimes only a biopsy can distinguish it from Crohn's. Biopsy means taking a sample of the gut lining and examining it under the microscope.
- Acute appendicitis, as in Eileen's case.
- Peptic ulcer.

- Bowel cancer.
- Abdominal tuberculosis.

Fortunately there are various tests and investigations, particularly special types of X-ray and endoscopy, and sometimes ultrasound, to help doctors to make sure they have the right diagnosis (see Chapter 7). Several conditions may crop up in the course of Crohn's with symptoms outside the digestive system. It is important to recognize these as related to the Crohn's process, and deal with them accordingly. Examples are arthritis, including severe back problems, conjunctivitis and other eye disorders, and various skin troubles. These are dealt with in detail in Chapter 6.

4

Children and adolescents

The proportion of youngsters, even babies, developing Crohn's has been increasing ever since the disease was recognized. Nowadays about a third of cases are diagnosed before the age of 21, with 12 per cent under 15. Official statistics always lag behind events, but we know that in 1974 ten children in every 100,000 developed Crohn's each year in the UK, and that this was four times as many as in 1959. Those living in this country who are most at risk are Afro-Caribbean, Indian and Jewish children. Just as with adults, Crohn's is most prevalent among youngsters living in urban industrial settings.

The special, defining characteristic of childhood Crohn's is the disruption of growth and development, due almost entirely to lack of nourishment.

How the illness may be recognized in children

Failure to grow at the normal rate

As in adults, Crohn's disease usually comes to notice because of abdominal pain, diarrhoea and undernutrition, the last being the most important. While adults lose weight, in children there is, instead, a slowdown in their growth rate. This can easily go unnoticed for some time, or be dismissed with 'he's a late developer', especially as the abdominal symptoms may not appear at first. Kind friends and even doctors are liable to reassure worried parents that their child 'is growing at his or her own pace' and that puberty will eventually proceed normally and the lag in growth will correct itself. Partly because of this attitude, the diagnosis of Crohn's in children is delayed on average by three years from the onset of the first indications of the disorder. It is growth in height that is most severely affected and is the most obvious.

Once Crohn's disease has been suspected, the diagnosis can be clinched by X-rays or endoscopy (see Chapter 7).

Loss of weight

If undernutrition and failure to grow properly are allowed to continue, a child may begin to lose weight. This is a serious symptom in a child who should be growing.

Failure to develop sexually

If Crohn's starts up before puberty, sexual development is delayed. This can be very embarrassing for a youngster at school and, more importantly, if the sex organs remain immature for too long, the boy or girl will have difficulty forming teenage relationships and may be unable to have children later.

Crohn's of the mouth

Symptoms affecting the two ends of the digestive system, the mouth and the anus, occur more often in the young than in adults. Crohn's disease of the mouth is especially troublesome. There may be painful cracks, ulcers and fissures in the mucous membrane lining the mouth and, most distressing of all, swelling, ulceration and fissuring of the lips, the 'thick lip syndrome'. It seldom occurs in adults, while in children with Crohn's it is a frequent cause of refusal to eat – adding to the other causes of undernutrition.

Unfortunately the steroid ointments which are so effective in most skin disorders do very little for 'thick lip', but steroids by mouth can be helpful, if used with care (see p. 59). In extreme cases, where it is urgent to get some nourishment into the child, tube-feeding may be necessary (see Chapter 10).

Jamie

Jamie was 11 when he began saying he had a 'tummy ache' and having bouts of diarrhoea. He must have had 'silent' Crohn's for some time, because in spite of having quite tall parents, he was short for his age and showed no signs of approaching puberty. He was one of the unlucky ones who developed Crohn's of the mouth, oral Crohn's disease, and for a short period – before he had treatment – he could only take nourishment through a straw. Ointment was useless, but steroid medication by mouth helped both his oral and his abdominal symptoms to subside.

The snag for children is that steroid medicines, like Crohn's itself, hold back normal growth and cannot be used freely.

Jamie's Crohn's disease had come on at a time of family tension, when his parents were divorcing, but he slowly improved with treatment, when his home life, with his mother, became more settled. Both his parents were concerned about his sexually immature body, but when he had managed to take in a generous diet, with supplements, his delayed puberty was normal when it arrived. At 18 Jamie is only a little below average height and he has a very nice girlfriend.

Ano-rectal Crohn's

Symptoms affecting the back passage, ano-rectal Crohn's, are sometimes the first manifestation of Crohn's disease in children and especially adolescents. They may precede the classic small intestine disorder by several years. Perianal (round the anus) problems can be agonizingly embarrassing for those in the most sensitive period of their lives, teenagers. Leakage or discharge can be devastating to social activities and seriously inhibit the development of intimate relationships.

Saeed

Saeed, at 18, was his parents' pride and joy. From his inner city comprehensive he had obtained a place at a prestigious university – Cambridge – and was all set for a sparkling career in science. It more than made up for his lack of prowess in sport. To be honest, Saeed was something of a weed, undersized and without much physical staying power. It was when it became excruciatingly painful to pass a motion that he went reluctantly to the GP.

The doctor did not like what he saw and started asking Saeed about his sexual orientation and experience, and if anyone had interfered with him sexually when he was younger. He also suggested an interview with Saeed's father. Saeed felt insulted. His sexual apparatus, like the rest of him, was undersized and his interest in that direction was lukewarm. What the doctor had seen were a few untidy tags of swollen skin round Saeed's anus, which he had thought at first were signs of sexual abuse. This is a not uncommon mistake in such cases. However, the doctor referred Saeed to the hospital where the skin tags were recognized by a bright young registrar as one of the characteristics of ano-rectal Crohn's. Microscopic examination of a biopsy sample from one of the tags confirmed the diagnosis. Saeed had no symptoms elsewhere in his body, but his poor physique and sexual immaturity indicated that the disease had been present for years, causing long-term undernutrition.

A steroid ointment and metronidazole controlled Saeed's problem moderately well, but he will probably opt for a surgical solution later.

Up to 95 per cent of Crohn's sufferers find it preferable or necessary to have an operation sooner or later. The procedures are described in Chapter 8. When the diseased area has been removed, the child's – or adult's – quality of life takes an upturn which lasts. Children are naturals for adapting to new situations, and they cope well, for instance, with an *ileostomy*, in which a loop of the ileum is brought to the surface and acts like an anus.

Diffuse small intestine Crohn's disease

Although the young are especially prone to developing the disease in the mouth or back passage, more show the usual adult symptoms of pain and diarrhoea because of Crohn's of the intestines. Youngsters are unlucky in that nearly the whole of the ileum may be affected, *diffuse ileitis*, as opposed to the more common, patchy involvement. Diffuse small intestine Crohn's is found in 13 per cent of children, compared with 4 per cent of adults with Crohn's, while fewer children, proportionately, have the illness confined to the colon.

The result is an even more serious degree of undernutrition – at a stage in life when more, rather than less, nourishment is required. The younger the child the more important this is.

Factors which hold back growth

- Inflammation or infection anywhere, especially with a raised temperature.
- Eating less because of anorexia, or to avoid pain in the mouth or with passing a motion.
- Increased loss of nutrients from diarrhoea, vomiting, bleeding or the vicious circle effect of protein loss, leading to greater inability to absorb it.
- Catch-up growth followed by standstill.
- Growth hormone lack.
- Side-effects of certain medication, such as corticosteroids and sulphasalazine.
- In addition, if parents do not check their child's height and weight regularly or accurately, they may miss the downward trend – or, more likely, the standstill – of undernutrition.

Treatment in children and young people

The goals are:

- To suppress and then control the active disease.
- To get the child back on track with growth and development.
- To get enough nourishment into the child for all their needs, plus extra for catch-up growth, and for puberty itself.
- To avoid or reduce, as far as possible, unpleasant symptoms or feelings, hospital admissions, time off school.
- To minimize the side-effects of medicines the child has to take.

- To avoid or reduce the use of steroids.
- To build up the child's self-confidence and encourage normal pre-teen and teenage clothes, appearance, interests and activities with peer group.
- To hold surgical treatment in reserve for acute situations.

Specific treatment includes various medicines, used particularly with a view to avoid having to take steroids more often than on alternate days, the elemental diet (see p. 96) and other special diets with an emphasis on protein and calories in general, with supplements. Feeding may be given by a tube into the stomach or by a vein when urgent building-up is, required.

Steroids (corticosteroids)

These are the quickest and most effective medicines for halting the acute symptoms, but for children in particular they have special dangers which must be weighed against the benefits. As little as 5 mg of prednisolone daily is enough to suppress normal growth. The bones are at especial risk, and boys seem to be more susceptible than girls to a delay in the growing and maturing of the skeleton. There is a shortage of calcium (osteopenia) in the vertebrae which constitute the backbone. Long-term or continuous use of steroids must be avoided in children. See Chapter 8 on treatment.

The outlook for your child

Although they can be acutely ill for a variable period, very few children die from Crohn's disease. What you can expect is a stormy period – illness-wise – around puberty, in addition to the normal early teenage ructions. Calmer waters follow. Although most children, like other Crohn's patients, will require surgery at some time in their lives, they do not have the same propensity that adults have for repeated severe attacks.

The absolutely vital element in managing Crohn's disease in a child is the attitude of the parents. The youngsters are bound to have emotional setbacks, frustrations and disappointments at school and among their friends. They must learn to live with Crohn's and cope with the rough-and-tumble of life. They may find over-concerned, over-protective parents undermining. An anxiously hovering mum can do more harm than good by confirming how difficult life is with Crohn's, and how fraught with dangers. As a parent you must steel yourself not to show signs of worry, but to accept risk-taking and applaud all social activities which show the independence of the younger generation.

The symptoms of Crohn's are, by their nature, infantilizing. You must do all you can to counteract this even if this means withholding help when you ache to give it, and not allowing too close a relationship to develop between you and your child. Independence is precious; it comes from having to manage for oneself at a level just past what seems possible. No other way stretches both capabilities and confidence.

Professional help

Counselling or skilled psychotherapy can help your child through a bumpy patch, probably at puberty or in adolescent years when relationships loom large. Interrupted schooling may mean extra study is needed with a tutor – not a parent – although many youngsters with Crohn's achieve their full academic potential without any help.

Tilly

Tilly and her brother Nat both developed Crohn's in the same year, although he was ten years older (their parents had had fertility problems between the two births). Nat was 24 and living with his girlfriend when the bouts of diarrhoea and vomiting began. Tilly was only 14, and rather fed up. All the other girls were having periods and wearing bras, while she remained small and dainty – and child-like. Partly because she was not distracted by a burgeoning interest in boys, she did particularly well at her studies.

If it had not been for the tummy aches, and increasingly often feeling sick and generally unwell and exhausted, you would have expected her to do brilliantly well when it came to GCSEs and all that follows. But by that time – she was 16 – she was seriously worried about having no periods and hardly any figure. She was still only 4 ft 10 ins, and had been that height for ages. No one suspected Crohn's disease at first, but one of the abdominal X-rays provided the first clue.

Tilly was very much into everything organic and natural, so she showed great determination in persisting with the unpalatable elemental diet for weeks, and later a less restricted one which avoided all dairy products. She has done well – with no steroids – and only has to go back on the elemental diet for three or four weeks at a time when the symptoms creep back.

5

The over-sixties

Crohn's disease is typically a young adults' illness. In fact, it was not until the 1950s, a quarter of a century after it was recognized and named, that anyone realized that it could affect people who were over 50, let alone those in their sixties or even more senior. Today, 10 per cent of those newly diagnosed with Crohn's are over 50, and there are more women than men among them.

Until very recently, it has been almost impossible to distinguish between Crohn's and the other IBD, ulcerative colitis, in this age group, particularly since Crohn's in the elderly occurs in the colon rather than the ileum. The diagnosis used to be in doubt in up to 20 per cent of cases, but this is improving. The symptoms are much the same in both illnesses and the naked eye appearance of the lining of the intestine is similar, with thickening, ulceration and deep fissures. It is the advent of the fibreoptic endoscope that has made accurate diagnosis feasible. This flexible instrument allows the doctor to see round corners, and take samples of tissue for microscopical examination. Examination by this method is called endoscopy or, more specifically, colonoscopy. It is quite a tricky procedure, however, compared with the older method of passing a shorter, rigid tube called a sigmoidoscope into the back passage.

Now that doctors are diagnosing Crohn's disease across the whole age range, it is becoming clear that there are two peaks in the incidence of the disease (*incidence* refers to the number of new cases cropping up each year). The two peak age groups are 20 to 29 and 70 to 79. In the older age group, there is a possibility that another condition, *ischaemic colitis*, may be clouding the issue. In older people the little arteries supplying blood to the lining of the large intestine sometimes get furred up. With poor circulation the tissues are subject to ulceration and inflammation, resulting in diarrhoea and bleeding. It may be that some people diagnosed as having Crohn's are really suffering from ischaemic colitis. Like so much about Crohn's disease, the jury is still out.

The over-sixties with Crohn's react differently from younger adults, not in the type of symptoms but in their severity. On the whole, older people fare better.

- They have fewer complaints of bad pain, by about 30 per cent.
- There is less likelihood, by 75 per cent, of sizeable lumps of inflamed tissue (*granulomas*) developing.

- They have less diarrhoea.
- By contrast, they are three times more likely to have bleeding from the back passage.
- The ileum is 30 per cent less likely to be affected.
- The colon, particularly the lower part, the storage section, is more likely to be involved.
- The left side of the abdomen is affected in 40 per cent of older sufferers, compared with younger people in whom the right side is nearly always the site of any pain.

One disadvantage of the symptoms being milder in the elderly is that with their tendency not to complain, not to 'bother the doctor', the time-lag between the first symptoms and diagnosis is unnecessarily long. Valuable time is wasted, with the risk of complications developing, including obstruction and bowel cancer.

The leading symptoms

- Diarrhoea is the commonest symptom, but is not usually as severe as in other age groups.
- Loss of weight is the second commonest, but you are less likely to notice your clothes getting looser than getting too tight, so a regular weigh-in is good policy.
- Abdominal discomfort, running into pain, is the third commonest symptom.
- Raised temperature occurs more often than in younger people.
- Copious bleeding from the rectum is typical of the older Crohn's sufferer, with an increased likelihood of anaemia as a result.
- The part round the anus – the perianal area – is involved more often than in younger adults, but not as severely as among the adolescents (see pp. 32, 76).

Because the symptoms are often milder in the over-sixties, and they are apt to assume that they must accept some imperfections of bodily function as they grow older, it can happen that the first time the person with Crohn's consults their doctor is in an emergency. For instance, the ulceration may have penetrated the wall of the colon and set off peritonitis in the covering membranes. Or acute obstruction of the bowel, particularly the small bowel, may occur. In either of these situations there is severe pain, and often collapse, and the victim must be rushed to hospital for intensive treatment.

Diverticular disease

This is a very common wear-and-tear disorder of the colon, affecting 30 per cent of the over-sixties. The intestinal wall becomes weaker after the age of fifty, like other parts of the body. Weak spots in the colon walls bulge into little pouches called *diverticula*, a condition known as *diverticulosis*. Naturally enough, some of the bowel contents, which have now become faeces or motions, get caught up. They may set up painful inflammation and infection in the gut lining – *diverticulitis*. There may be some bleeding, but not as bad as in Crohn's.

Diverticular disease is unpleasant in its own right, but not dangerous. The big danger is that the doctor may put the symptoms of Crohn's down to this relatively unimportant condition, delaying proper diagnosis. To confuse the issue further, Crohn's frequently develops in a part of the colon already affected by diverticular disease.

Philippa

Philippa, aged 66, had always had trouble with her bowels. She had a tendency to constipation for which she had taken various laxatives for years. Her doctor was one of those who believe such a habit predisposes the colon to develop Crohn's disease, cancer, or the much commoner, less important diverticular disease. It was when she was 62 that Philippa began to have what was unusual for her – loose motions. She had bouts of diarrhoea with blood and mucus, with abdominal discomfort, just short of pain. Reasonably enough, her doctor assumed she had the common, recurrent condition of infected diverticula – diverticulitis. He prescribed antibiotics, but they did no good. The condition rumbled on.

Good periods alternated with the episodes of diarrhoea. The GP began to have doubts about the diagnosis and was anxious not to miss a serious illness. He sent off a blood test which showed that Philippa had a haemoglobin level of 7.8 g/dl (the normal range for a woman is 11.5–16.5 g/dl), indicating anaemia. She also had a low level of albumin (26 g/l instead of 36–47), and a high white blood cell count. These results pointed to active disease and were consistent with Crohn's. The hospital specialist, Philippa's next port of call, settled the matter with a colonoscopy. Philippa had Crohn's disease. She responded well to medicines for her anaemia and her Crohn's disease, respectively, plus a high-protein, high calorie diet.

It is vitally important to recognize and begin the treatment of Crohn's promptly in the elderly, even more so than in younger adults. Older people are more susceptible to serious complications, such as toxic dilatation of the colon, perforation (a break in the intestinal wall), septicaemia, or severe haemorrhage causing a dangerous drop in the volume of circulating blood. This disrupts the essential working of the heart and lungs (see Chapter 6).

Points to look out for

Crohn's disease is likely to be a long, smouldering illness, with loss of weight, while diverticular disease presents itself in recurrent acute attacks of abdominal pain, without weight loss, and without the general malaise of Crohn's. Bleeding from the rectum is more severe in Crohn's, with anaemia a likely result. The symptoms of anaemia itself are often vague, but they include weakness, fatigue, shortness of breath, dizziness, headache, tinnitus, insomnia and swollen ankles.

The other disorder which often gets confused with Crohn's is ischaemic colitis. This differs from Crohn's in coming on suddenly, often in a person who already has some heart, blood pressure or circulatory problem. Bleeding or clotting problems after operations of any kind are likely in people who are susceptible to ischaemic colitis, while the inflammatory lumps of granulomatous tissue characteristic of Crohn's are never present in this disorder.

The outlook

This is better in Crohn's if you are elderly to start with. You stand a 42 per cent chance of requiring surgery, which is a good deal less than in younger patients, and in those suffering from ulcerative colitis. What is most cheering is that the prognosis for seniors with Crohn's has improved enormously over the last few years. This is largely because of earlier, more accurate diagnosis, so that appropriate management is begun sooner. Even a barium X-ray to show the outline of the colon often revealed only the bulges of diverticular disease, and Crohn's went unrecognized. Endoscopy and biopsy (see pp. 52, 53) put the correct answer beyond doubt.

Treatment also has improved in the life-threatening situations, not so much because of the drugs, but with better tube-feeding or intravenous nourishment, more sophisticated modern methods of intensive care and new – safer – surgery. Chapter 8 describes in detail the medical and surgical treatments. They are just as effective in older sufferers as in other age groups.

Paul

Paul had retired from his merchant banking firm nearly ten years before and was concentrating on his golf. He had been the club captain twice. At 70 he had never had a major illness and his only operation had been for a hernia. Apart from a slight fall-off in energy he was as well as ever. He had what he called 'the colly-wobbles' occasionally: noisy gurgling in his abdomen and mild colicky pains which did not last. So he was unprepared for the night when he woke at 2 a.m., vomited several times and had one bowel movement, and the most excruciating colicky pains in the middle of his abdomen.

The locum GP diagnosed obstruction and Paul was whisked off to hospital. The GP had been right, and the obstruction proved to be due to a stricture (narrowing) in his small intestine near the junction with the caecum. The surgeon removed the affected part and constructed an ileostomy – an opening on the surface, from the healthy part of the ileum. Paul recovered well from the operation and has become good friends with his ileostomy nurse.

He is thinking of trying nine holes very soon.

6

Effects outside the digestive system

You would not guess that a teenager with a painful ankle was showing the first sign of Crohn's disease, or that the lumps that came up, out of the blue, on Pat's shins could be anything to do with an illness in her small intestine. Yet they were.

Almost any bodily system can be caught up in the Crohn's process, probably through an ill-understood immunity reaction. These 'off-piste' symptoms are important, not only because they are unpleasant in themselves and require treatment, but because they may alert you – or your doctor – to the possibility of Crohn's disease. They can make you take notice of any mild bowel symptoms you might have ignored until then, and stimulate your doctor to run some tests.

Skin disorders

These are the most obvious. There are three types associated with Crohn's, all with impressive names: *erythema nodosum*, which are the lumps that Pat had (see below), its cousin *erythema multiforme*, and *pyoderma gangrenosum*. Erythema multiforme consists of raised lumps often of a target shape, blistering in the middle, but with no fixed pattern. Pyoderma gangrenosum is the most serious and it only occurs in Crohn's or the other IBD, ulcerative colitis. It begins with a batch of spots, full of pus like boils, which break down to form ulcers. They are caused by a common germ, the staphylococcus, and the first line of treatment is with antibiotics.

Pat
Pat was 29. She often had tummy aches and the squits, and the possibility of Crohn's disease or ulcerative colitis had been mooted but never followed up. Then these painful, dusky, purplish-red lumps appeared on her legs, and she felt ill into the bargain – as though she had 'flu. All her joints ached, she had a temperature and she could not face food. Her GP recognized the characteristic skin reaction of erythema nodosum. The possible causes were the contraceptive pill, chlamydia, various infections – and IBD.

Pat had to stay in bed for a week, but it was a month before the lumps went down, leaving what looked like bruises which lasted several more weeks. By that time, with what Pat could tell him, the doctor had worked out that she had IBD. The small dose of a steroid that she was given for her bowels chased off the skin problem at the same time.

Arthritis

Arthritis is the disorder most frequently encountered outside the digestive system in Crohn's disease. Sometimes – in about half the cases – the pain, *arthralgia*, is present in the joints, but there is no inflammation nor any abnormality in an X-ray. The joints most commonly affected are the hips and ankles, perhaps because they are subject to the stresses of weight-bearing. The sacro-iliac joints, at the bottom of the back, or the back itself, can also be affected. A particularly disabling back disorder, *ankylosing spondylitis*, can occur with Crohn's, but fortunately it is rare.

Zoe

Zoe was 15, a weedy type, and lately always complaining that she was tired. She had a minute appetite and everyone thought this was a slimming ploy. While her friends were gradually filling out their bras and girdles and getting taller, Zoe was as flat as a lath and losing weight. It was all put down to her finicky refusal to eat properly. Her periods had not kicked in yet but a late start was a family trait, so no one was greatly concerned.

Now Zoe started saying that she could not walk because her hip joints hurt. X-rays showed nothing so she was shunted off to a child guidance clinic. She gave up complaining, so perhaps the discussions had helped. Anyway, it was not until seven months later that the colicky abdominal pains began. This time the investigations included a special type of X-ray, with a barium meal, a drink which shows up as it passes down the alimentary canal. This showed the 'string sign' – a very much narrowed segment of the small intestine, representing an area of spasm in the muscles of its wall, and a dead give-away for Crohn's disease.

With the diagnosis made, Zoe was given the appropriate treatment. After a brief boost with a steroid to start things off, she took a drug called sulphasalazine and as much nourishment as she could manage. The hope is that there is enough growth potential left in her long bones for her to make up for the period of snail-pace development.

Anaemia

Anaemia is commonplace, practically routine, in Crohn's disease, especially the simple type due to iron deficiency. If the small intestine is not functioning properly, iron, among other important minerals and vitamins, cannot be absorbed. If, on the other hand, the colon is the part of the gut most affected, bleeding from the ulcerated areas leads to the same result. The body normally recycles its iron so that when red blood corpuscles are discarded, usually when they are about six weeks old, the iron is salvaged for the new replacement cells. When there is bleeding for any reason the iron is lost together with all the other constituents of the blood.

There is another kind of anaemia which crops up rather less often in Crohn's disease: *autoimmune haemolytic anaemia*. Autoimmune refers to a mistake made by the immune system, so that it attacks and tries to destroy some of its own cells as though they were invaders. In this case, it is the red blood cells that are picked on. Haemolytic means blood-destroying. In haemolytic anaemia the pigment from the cells is released into the fluid part of the blood, the plasma, and shows up yellowish in the skin, the membranes and the white part of the eyes. Finally it is taken up into the urine, making this a darker colour than usual.

Faulty working of the immune system is an ill-understood part of Crohn's which may result in this type of anaemia. When red blood cells have been destroyed replacements cannot be manufactured properly if there is a shortage, through malabsorption, of vitamins B12 and folate. This compounds the situation. There is also the *hypochromic anaemia* of chronic diseases in general. The appearance under the microscope of the blood looks just like iron-deficiency anaemia, but the iron stores are well stocked – there seems to be a block on using it.

The main symptoms of anaemia, such as fatigue, pallor and shortness of breath, are common to all three types.

Colin

Colin Chan came to the UK from Hong Kong at the time of the handover and managed to land an administrative job in a Birmingham hospital. He was 32 and had high hopes for his future. The snag was that, ridiculous as it seemed at his age, he was slowing down. Everything took twice as long and seemed such an effort. He was puffed when he played tennis and could feel his heart thumping away. He was also having pains in the lower right hand corner of his abdomen and had lost his appetite. Sometimes he had a throbbing headache – not the tension kind – and although he felt exhausted he could not sleep. Once or twice he felt quite dizzy and thought he might faint.

It was when the ringing in his ears started that he decided to ask a doctor friend at the hospital to check him over and to see whether there was anything wrong, or if he was just a hypochondriac. Colin's friend did not pick up the slight yellowing of the whites of his eyes and skin, nor think to ask about the colour of his urine, so jaundice did not figure in his mind. However, he did arrange a blood test and found that Colin had a mix of two kinds of anaemia. He had deficiencies of iron, and of the vitamins B12 and folic acid.

It was then that the young doctor homed in on the two symptoms which were not due to anaemia: the pain in the appendix area and the loss of appetite. The complete picture emerged: Crohn's disease causing malabsorption, causing anaemia. Colin had to have dietary supplements, and he also had a stricturoplasty, a repair of a diseased part of the ileum which was in danger of blockage. Azathioprine was the non-steroidal medication chosen to control the Crohn's after that.

Colin had a number of the usual symptoms of anaemia, but he missed out on chest pains (*angina*), swelling ankles (*oedema*), poor vision, a raised heart rate, and pins and needles in the fingers and toes.

Eye disorders

Inflammation of the eye is another unexpected concomitant of Crohn's disease. Any part of the eye may be affected.

Stephen
Stephen blamed the sore, gritty feel in his eyes on staring at a VDU so much of the time. He had conjunctivitis, inflammation of the 'skin' covering the front of the eye. His Crohn's disease had been in remission for several months but there had recently been a very stressful period at work, with a new boss who wanted everything done differently. The conjunctivitis was the first indication of a relapse, with more frequent motions and a mild fever in the evenings. An increase in Stephen's medication and a few sessions of counselling helped to ward off a more serious attack.

Conjunctivitis like Stephen's is the simplest and least serious, but other eye disorders which may be associated with Crohn's disease include *uveitis, episcleritis, keratitis, retinitis* and *retrobulbar neuritis* – each being inflammation in one or other part of the eye. Any discomfort in the eyes or impairment of vision needs expert attention but also serves as a reminder to review your current treatment and lifestyle, if you have established Crohn's disease.

Heart and blood vessels

The heart and blood vessels may seem a far cry from intestinal illness but any blood vessel, from the big arteries and veins down to the tiniest capillaries may react to Crohn's disease (and some other chronic conditions) by inflammation. This is called *vasculitis*, and one theory is that vasculitis of the small vessels in the gut wall underlies the tendency to ulceration. Some people with Crohn's develop *pericarditis* or *myocarditis*, inflammation of the membrane enclosing the heart and the heart muscle itself, respectively. The symptoms are chest pain, shortness of breath and faints.

Liver and gall bladder

There are a number of problems in this area which may be an indirect result of Crohn's disease. Cholesterol gallstones are common, but especially so in Crohn's, from middle age onwards. They only cause trouble if one stone gets wedged in the bile duct. This can set off inflammation of the whole gall bladder/bile duct system.

Aaron
Aaron was 53. He had coped with Crohn's disease for eight years and felt he had it taped when he was woken up, out of the blue, at 2 a.m., by an agonizingly sharp pain high up in his abdomen. He thought it was due to a cholesterol-rich birthday dinner he had enjoyed with his family that evening. It had featured goulash and a luscious cream sweet and may indeed have been the stimulus to extra activity in the digestive system.

The pain was not colicky, but continued at full strength all the time. When the doctor arrived, bleary-eyed, it had shifted slightly to the right and even Aaron's shoulder hurt on that side. Then he started vomiting and his temperature rocketed. In the hospital X-rays and ultrasound showed up the gallstones. Aaron was given a morphine injection for the pain, and a drip to top up his fluid level. When the acute symptoms settled, the question of surgery came up. The Crohn's was no bar to that.

A much rarer disorder is *sclerosing cholangitis*, an inflammation of the bile duct with narrowing from scar tissue, much like stricture-formation in Crohn's ileitis (inflammation of the ileum). Cholangitis nearly always arises in Crohn's disease, and ulcerative colitis, the other IBD. It does not come on suddenly like gallstone pain, but shows up first with jaundice and fever which come and go, and pain in the same area as gall bladder pain. Often the skin itches – all over. Antibiotics help, but steroids are no use.

Cirrhosis of the liver has a reputation for being associated with alcohol, and it often is, but teetotal Crohn's patients can also develop it. The liver, in the right upper abdomen, at first enlarges with fat, then shrinks and becomes knobbly as scar tissue forms. Cirrhosis is more dangerous than Crohn's disease.

Gordon

Gordon was 34. He had had Crohn's since he was 19. His work as a freelance journalist meant that many of the best assignments seemed to be handed out in a bar, not that he was by any means a heavy drinker, unlike some of his colleagues. Gradually Gordon was becoming aware of vague discomfort in his upper abdomen, different from the pain low down on the right which he felt when his Crohn's was playing up. Otherwise there was nothing that the Crohn's might not account for: tiredness, weakness, loss of appetite with nausea, bloating and loss of weight (it was falling off him now). There was nothing specific about any of these symptoms.

It was not until he came off his motorbike that he had a chat with his GP. Gordon had not suffered any bony injury but there was extensive bruising. He told the doctor as a matter of interest that he bruised very easily these days and mentioned that he 'hadn't been feeling too great', what with the discomfort in his abdomen. The doctor found a place that was tender when he pressed it, under Gordon's ribs on the right, and he ran a few blood tests. They showed that his liver was not functioning properly, possibly the beginning of cirrhosis. Some of his journalist friends had come to grief that way, so he was scared enough to take it seriously when he was told that he must give up alcohol altogether if he was to have a long life.

Since he was not addicted, Gordon was able to stick to the veto, and he also followed – under advice – a totally re-arranged diet, low in fat but high in protein and carbohydrate, with supplements of the vitamins B12, C, D and folic acid, and calcium. After three months his liver function tests were near normal. Fatty liver – the final diagnosis – is fairly common in Crohn's but is recoverable with strict attention to diet and a lifestyle without alcohol.

Urinary system

This is no more immune than other parts from the effects of Crohn's disease. Sometimes one of the swollen parts of the ileum can press on one of the ureters, the twin tubes which convey the urine from the kidneys to the bladder. If the urine cannot flow down freely on one side there is back pressure on that kidney, causing pain in the small of the back. There is danger of infection setting in, with sudden pain in the loin, radiating round to the front, vomiting and high fever. Antibiotic treatment is urgent.

Edmund had a very different water problem.

Edmund

Edmund had been a Crohn's sufferer for six years and had managed fairly well with several medicines. He was 39 when he started having bladder infections, one after another – fairly unusual for a man. Antibiotics helped, but not for long: it was a miserable situation. What took him by surprise was that he seemed to be passing bubbles of air in his water. When it happened again his GP referred him to a urogenital surgeon. Examination with a cystoscope, an instrument for looking inside the bladder, provided the answer – a fistula coming through from the colon. An operation was required to remove the offending piece of colon, ulcerated through by Crohn's, and the bladder was repaired. It healed within two weeks and Edmund has had no urinary infections since. No bladder could have stood up to a constant leakage of material from the colon.

One residual problem was Edmund's dip into depression, with low mood, poor sleep and loss of appetite. With Crohn's he could not afford to lose any more weight, so after he left the surgical ward, he spent six weeks as a day patient in the psychiatric department, his treatment involving a mix of individual cognitive therapy, various group therapies, including one for drama, and an antidepressant.

The respiratory system

The respiratory system is affected in as many as 30 per cent of those with Crohn's disease, but usually the symptoms are too mild to be troublesome. The lung may react to Crohn's with what is called *alveolitis*, an inflammation of the small, delicate air sacs which comprise the lung tissue. If a significant number are involved you may develop a persistent, dry cough and become short of breath with exercise.

A chest X-ray will reveal the problem and treatment is much the same as for Crohn's itself: the steroid prednisolone backed up by azathioprine, to reduce the need for a large dose of the steroid.

Metastatic Crohn's disease

All the conditions described so far as linked with Crohn's disease, but outside the digestive system, have arisen as a reaction to the intestinal illness in one way or another. Metastatic Crohn's disease is different. It *is* Crohn's disease. Patches of typical Crohn's inflammation appear somewhere unconnected with any other affected area – it is not a matter of simple spread. Any part of the skin may show Crohn's-type swelling, redness and ulceration, but most often it is below the waist, for instance at the navel or on the thigh. The genitals and the skin between them and the anus are quite often involved.

One young fellow accepted his Crohn's with good grace until a strange sore place appeared on his penis. He went to the special clinic, furious to think that his trusted partner had infected him with an STD (sexually transmitted disease). None of the usual infections in that area were responsible, but a sample (biopsy) of the skin showed unmistakable Crohn's and a few ordinary skin bacteria. Fortunately, the sore patch responded to a steroid cream. He had to apologize to his girlfriend.

Of course you will not get all of these unpleasant symptoms; in fact you may not be affected by any of them, but it may be helpful to be aware of them and realize that they could be connected with your Crohn's disease.

7

Finding out: investigations

You have symptoms you want to be rid of, and they could be due to Crohn's disease – or one of several other disorders. Before any treatment can begin, your doctor needs to find out for sure which one it is.

To start the diagnostic hunt he or she will want to hear about the information your body itself is providing in the form of symptoms, such as pain, loose motions and losing weight. How long you have had them, and have you any idea what set them off? Have you had anything similar before, and if so, what happened? If any of your relatives have had bowel problems, what was the diagnosis?

The physical examination may reveal a tender place in the appendix area, and your doctor may be able to feel a definite lump of inflamed tissue. He or she will also be able to judge if you have recently lost weight and whether you have the general pallor of skin and membranes to indicate anaemia.

After the examination and answering all the questions, you will probably be asked to provide a specimen of your motions – the receptacle will be provided. A pale, frothy motion means malabsorption, evidence that your small intestine is not working properly. If there is blood and mucus in the sample it indicates that the colon is inflamed and ulcerated, but if bleeding occurs in the small intestine, which is less common, the motions are black and tarry. Part of the specimen will be sent to the laboratory for culture, to find what bacteria will grow and to test which antibiotics are effective against them. There will be a heavier growth of bacteria than normal in Crohn's, but unfortunately the chief suspect, mycobacterium paratuberculosis (Mptb for short) is extremely slow and difficult to grow in culture. In a recent research study it took between 13 and 40 months. This is obviously no help in diagnosing what is wrong with someone who is suffering today.

Identifying the particular mycobacterium has also presented major problems, but the development of DNA probes promises useful results (see Chapter 12).

Another big snag is that the abdomen keeps its secrets hidden. You cannot tell from the outside what is going on inside – any more than you can tell by looking at the outside of someone's house what they are doing within. Fortunately, technology has come to the rescue and brought some of the secrets of abdominal disorders out of the realms of guesswork. A whole range of techniques is now available for detecting and assessing Crohn's disease.

Radiology

X-rays were first used in the investigation of Crohn's in 1934, only two years after it was recognized as an illness. The intestines do not show up in X-rays so they need to be outlined by a material that is opaque to them. A suspension of barium is harmless and shows up well. It is routinely used in so-called barium 'meals' and enemas. An extra refinement is to introduce air or gas into the part to be visualized. This appears black in contrast to the white produced by barium, and the combination is called *double-contrast radiology*.

Barium meal and follow-through

Before you begin you need to have your stomach and intestines empty – a matter of fasting, as for an operation, but the examination requires only out-patient attendance. The meal consists of a glass of white liquid, usually flavoured with peppermint. You swallow it slowly and the progress of the barium can be tracked by X-rays down the alimentary tract. While this method is still in use, it has been superseded by enteroclysis (see below) in some centres.

Enteroclysis

An improvement, in that it provides more and clearer detail, is the infusion of the suspension of barium directly into the intestine through a tube. This is called *enteroclysis*.

Even the tiny aphthoid ulcers in the lining of the gut can be seen with this method. Crops of these in the small intestine are probably the first visible sign of Crohn's. Larger ulcers develop later, with the general thickening of the gut wall. Greatly narrowed segments, the 'string sign', are especially characteristic of the disease. They are caused by spasm of the gut muscles. Cobblestone patterning occurs only in severe Crohn's. An irregular arrangement of patches of inflammation is another strong indication of Crohn's. 'Skip' lesions are patches like islands of inflammation in a sea of normal tissue, as though the disease had missed out or skipped some areas. All or some of these may be recognizable in a barium X-ray and support a diagnosis of Crohn's affecting the small intestine.

An interesting and characteristic effect of malabsorption is the clumping of the barium suspension in the ileum, due to an excess of digestive juices.

These X-rays may also pick up some common complications – sinuses and fistulas. Sinuses are ulcerated tracks that go through the full thickness of the gut wall, and in fistulas the ulceration extends into some other organ. Barium X-rays, particularly those from enteroclysis in expert hands, give valuable information for diagnosis and also in pinpointing the site of the problem when surgery is contemplated for obstruction or a fistula.

Howard

Howard was 24 when he started a new job in sales for a company making scientific instruments. It meant he spent a lot of his day travelling from one laboratory to another. He felt perfectly well apart from the inconvenience of having to find the loo so often, for his bowels. That and feeling tired – and losing weight. His home was in one of the most beautiful counties in England, and his local hospital was friendly and welcoming. The physician whom Howard saw there suspected Crohn's disease as soon as he heard Howard's story and he fixed up a barium meal and follow-through straightaway.

Howard found the experience not unpleasant, and very interesting, especially when the doctor explained the relevant X-rays to him. He showed him two features that pointed directly to Crohn's – the 'string' sign of a very narrow segment of gut and the flocculation (or clumping) of the barium. Patches of swollen mucous membrane could also be detected in the small intestine, and a few in the first part of the colon.

Howard's Crohn's was mild. He had ten days off work for rest and treatment. Then, with some rearrangement of his work schedule, to allow for reasonable breaks, and a re-jigging of his diet (his girlfriend was delighted with the changes) he remained well – and needed only a non-steroidal medicine.

Barium enema

The large intestine is best investigated by a barium enema. In essence, this is like any other enema except for the preliminaries. First there is the ordinary examination of the back passage with a gloved finger, then a *sigmoidoscopy*, usually a few days before the enema (see below). Since the bowel must be clean and clear for this special enema, you are given laxatives and a cleansing washout. Finally you are ready for the barium enema, often used in conjunction with air to stretch the colon lining for a better picture. The enema itself, including taking X-rays, takes only 25 to 30 minutes, but older people and those with heart complaints can find the whole procedure rather exhausting. Aim to rest afterwards.

CT scanning (computerized tomography)

This is a different kind of X-ray. It provides a series of shadow pictures of the body as though it were cut in slices one centimetre apart. The big advantage is that the organs surrounding the intestine can also be seen. CT scans are particularly valuable for Crohn's in the lowest parts of the alimentary tract, the rectum and around the anus, as barium enemas and follow-throughs do not provide a comprehensible picture in this area.

CT scans are of great help to surgeons in 'fistula mapping', where it is essential to know the way the muscles and other organs lie in relation to an ulcerated part – and they have a 90 per cent success rate in detecting fistulas involving the bladder (see Edmund, p. 47).

Endoscopy

This means 'inside looking' and is the second most frequently used investigative technique. The oldest and simplest method is sigmoidoscopy, in which an instrument with a light at the end, the sigmoidoscope, is passed into the back passage. It may be a rigid tube, or more recently, a flexible type. It gives a good view of the rectum and sometimes detects an inflamed, ulcerated area which the barium enema has missed. It is an advantage for the doctor actually to see the lining of the intestine, as opposed to mere outlines and shadows.

Colonoscopy and ileocolonoscopy

With the wonderful advances in fibreoptic technology, it is now possible to see the full length of the colon, to the caecum, with a colonoscope, and even further, into the ileum – ileocolonoscopy. The trick of fibreoptics is that whatever the instrument can 'see' at its tip is conveyed along the fibres, however long and tortuous their course through the intestines to the operator. It grants us the gift of seeing round corners.

The doctor is looking out for:

- Redness and perhaps bleeding from the lining membrane.
- Cobblestoning – the rough, irregular, knobbly pattern made by deep cracks dividing up the swollen, oedematous tissue (see p. 28).
- Ulcers. They may be tiny, white, pinhead aphthoid ulcers, with a red base; a deep, punched-out type, sometimes likened to a well; 'railroad track' ulcers running in straight lines; or the serpiginous kind in all sorts of shapes.
- Stenosis – narrowing from any cause. The ileocolonoscope can be slim enough to be passed gently into the narrow part to discover whether it

has a generally swollen or lumpy lining, or if tough, fibrous scarring is constricting the passage – or if something outside the intestine is pressing on it.

- Pseudopolyps – small tags of inflamed, swollen lining membrane intestine protruding like fingers. Usually they are unmistakable, but if there is any doubt that they may be true polyps, a *biopsy* is easily done.

Another brilliant facility of the fibreoptic endoscope is that it can take minute samples of tissue – biopsies – for microscopical examination. You can imagine how useful and reassuring it can be to be able to check that an odd, lumpy bit is not cancer but Crohn's.

Colonoscopy and ileocolonoscopy are the Rolls Royce of investigation methods in Crohn's, requiring a high degree of skill and experience, and they are available only in specialist centres. Barium X-rays are a trustworthy fall-back if you find yourself far from a big city.

Other types of endoscopy are used in other areas. If you have symptoms relating to your stomach or duodenum, *gastroscopy* or *duodenoscopy*, respectively, are the standard ploys for assessing the situation. On the rare occasions when the oesophagus seems to be the site of Crohn's symptoms, a simple, rigid *oesophagoscope* can be slipped in. A mild, muscle-relaxant sedative, like diazepam, takes the edge off any anxiety and discomfort during these procedures.

Ultrasound and endosonography

Ultrasound is another form of investigation into what is going on under wraps. Inaudible (to us) sound waves are directed towards the part to be examined, and measured as they bounce back, or echo, producing a black and white image. The whole process is filmed, with stills as necessary, and is most familiar from its routine use in pregnancy. Endosonography means that for greater precision the *echoprobe* which emits and picks up the sound waves is put inside the rectum.

Endosonography (ES) is most useful when there is an abscess or a fistula in the pelvic area which is particularly difficult to 'see' by other methods. It is important to know the exact location of either of these complications in relation to other vital structures in this crowded area, before active treatment is begun. ES is also employed to check the results of medical or surgical treatment before deciding on the next step. It is ideal to try simple rest and medicines first and check whether this is working before launching into complex surgery in a sensitive area.

Dorothy

Dorothy felt ill. She was 47 and had been on a roller-coaster of relapse and recovery for the last two years. Her Crohn's had come on originally when she was about 30, and although she had two or three bouts of illness she had always bounced back quite quickly. This time she continued to have a dragging pain in her pelvis and persistent fever. Passing a motion was agony.

Sigmoidoscopy and colonoscopy were not helpful, but echosonography with the scope in the vagina showed a cavity which did not produce an echo. It was an abscess, too low down for the other investigations. Dorothy was not keen on surgery, so she was treated medically. After three months another endosonograph showed that the abscess was definitely smaller, and by ten months it could no longer be seen. And Dorothy felt well.

Radio-labelled leucocyte scanning

Leucocytes are the white cells in the blood. Their major function is fighting infection; they are the foot soldiers in the battle, so many thousands are needed, including reserves which can be called upon when there is illness. They are transported in the bloodstream and, like passengers on a bus, stop off at the appropriate places.

In this type of scan a blood sample is taken from a vein. The white cells in it are 'labelled' with a short-life radio-active tag, and then returned to the circulation. Their progress can be followed with a gamma camera, which 'photographs' radiation. The white cells congregate in trouble spots within a few hours, pointing up areas of inflammation in both the small and large intestines at the same examination. The advantages of this kind of scanning are that it involves no risks, no special preparation and no more discomfort than two pinpricks, one to withdraw and one to return the blood sample. It can safely be used in someone who is severely ill, for whom colonoscopy or ileocolonoscopy would be dangerous.

Radio-labelled leucocyte scanning has been proved a more sensitive test for IBD than barium examinations, and provides a valuable objective assessment of how effective a particular treatment has been. It is at the forefront of modern investigative techniques, and research is actively taking place as you read.

Laboratory tests

Crohn's disease is an illness that fluctuates from the acute and incapacitating at one time to almost complete remission at another. It is useful to have some pointers to what is going on in the background. If you are in a bad phase, is it beginning to get better – or worse? If the illness is quiescent, what is the likelihood of relapse? Such considerations are particularly relevant if you are going through a period of emotional strain. Laboratory tests give your doctor factual information on which to base an anti-Crohn's strategy. It is helpful to have some idea what the results mean.

Active inflammation

This is reflected in two tests:

- The ESR (erythrocyte sedimentation rate) is higher than the normal 0–6 mm in one hour when there is infection or inflammation. More than 20 mm per hour shows a severe condition.
- The number of white blood cells (leucocytes) in your blood is raised above the normal 4,000–11,000 per microlitre (leucocytosis).

Anaemia

If you are anaemic the haemoglobin level in your blood is reduced. Normal levels are:

- 130–180 g/l for a man
- 115–165 g/l for a woman

Malabsorption

This is the result of the small intestine being unable to function properly. It may show in a shortage of certain minerals in your blood. The normal values are:

- calcium: 2.12–2.62 mmol/l
- magnesium: 0.75–1 mmol/l
- iron: 14–32 micromol/l for a man; 10–28 micromol/l for a woman
- zinc: 8–29 micromol/l

Other substances which may be inadequately absorbed in Crohn's are (normal values):

- vitamin B12: 160–925 nanograms/l (lacking in some forms of anaemia)
- folate: 6–21 micrograms/l (lacking in some forms of anaemia)
- albumin: 37–47 g/l (low in Crohn's because of poor absorption of proteins in general)

Special tests for malabsorption

- Fats: if these are not being absorbed properly from the ileum the motions will contain more than 7 grams of fat in 24 hours.
- Carbohydrates: lactose tolerance test and hydrogen breath test.

Evelyn

Evelyn, at 28, was due to get married. Like all Crohn's sufferers in her situation, she fretted about the sexual aspect. Suppose she was seized with uncontrollable diarrhoea at the critical moment, or one of her occasional periods of feverishness coincided with the honeymoon? They always seemed to come when she was anxious.

In the run-up to the day Evelyn's abdomen was a little tender and she was passing two or three motions a day – she tried to tell herself that it was only tension. Then her temperature began sneaking up to 38°C in the evenings. The doctor checked for active disease with an ESR and a blood count. They were both slightly out of the normal range. Evelyn asked if there was any way to ward off what seemed a mild – so far – threat of relapse at this stage. The doctor added a small dose of methylprednisolone to her non-steroidal medication, temporarily, but gave no promises. However, Evelyn sailed through the wedding and the honeymoon without mishap, and when they came back she had a check-up. Her raised ESR and leucocytosis (excess of white cells) had subsided.

Investigations in practice

The main point of investigations is to find out what is causing the unwelcome symptoms. Since different conditions require different kinds of treatment, it is important to get the answer right. The steps towards reaching a diagnosis begin with your complaints and may end with the ultimate: ileocolonoscopy and serial biopsies, with laboratory tests and X-rays en route. But no test is 100 per cent reliable.

Wendy

Wendy was 16 and in the middle of writing her A level English exam when a cramping pain in her abdomen doubled her up and a minute later she was flying to the loo with diarrhoea. The cramps and the diarrhoea, which poured out like water, persisted and Wendy felt sick and dizzy. No way could she continue with the English paper, so the invigilator sent her home in a taxi. She only vomited once, but she felt alternately boiling hot and freezing cold. When her mother came home from work she found Wendy in bed with all her clothes on and a temperature of 40°C.

The doctor took away a sample of the watery motion for culture and advised Wendy to drink as much as possible in the form of fruit-flavoured drinks and tea rather than plain water. He prescribed loperamide to control the diarrhoea, but no antibiotics at this stage, since they can make matters worse. The symptoms were slow to settle, and as the culture showed the presence of salmonella, he did give her some ciprofloxacillin, which is particularly effective against this infection. Even so, Wendy continued to have pain low in her abdomen and pass three or four motions a day.

An ileocolonoscopy showed shallow ulcers with red, inflamed edges in the lining of the colon on the left, and a cluster of aphthoid ulcers on the right. Under the microscope a small collection of granuloma cells could be seen. All of this was consistent with Crohn's disease, and at this point the diagnosis lay between this and salmonella colitis.

Six months later, a repeat ileocolonoscopy showed that all the ulcers had healed and both ileum and colon were clear. The microscopic appearances had reverted to normal, too. Crohn's disease was ruled out, and the final diagnosis was acute salmonella colitis, from which Wendy had recovered.

Martin

Martin was 18 when he went on a package holiday to Turkey where he had an attack of traveller's diarrhoea. At least that was what they thought. It started with twinges of pain in the appendix area, mild nausea and colic. When the diarrhoea started he went to a local pharmacist who suggested codeine phosphate to calm his bowels down. Since he was due to go home in a day or two, he decided to see his own doctor as soon as he got back. He was still having colicky pains and episodes of painful straining to pass small motions, streaked with blood and pus. The culture, when the result came back, showed a bug called shigelli flexneri, often a cause of dysentery. After a course of the appropriate antibiotic, Martin's symptoms began to subside, but within a few days they all came back and an ileocolonoscopy was done, to see what was going on.

The operator saw that Martin's colon was inflamed and had some shallow ulcers throughout its length; biopsies confirmed this. Martin's illness was labelled acute self-limited colitis – but it did not self-limit. It went on. Six months later, the doctor had to accept that Martin had chronic inflammatory bowel disease – probably Crohn's.

57

Even microscopical examination of a sample of the gut lining cannot provide a cast-iron guarantee of the correct diagnosis. Various intestinal infections can mimic IBD of the colon, but they do not affect the ileum, except possibly the last inch or so, where small and large intestine join.

In both these cases it was not until many months after the onset of the symptoms that the diagnosis could be made with certainty. Fortunately, with all the technical help available, this is exceptional.

8
Treatment

Part 1: Medicines

Crohn's disease is not an illness you just have to put up with – there is a range of treatments, and at different times you may need more than one of them:

- medicines
- surgery
- diet
- change in lifestyle
- psychological help

Whether you are feeling generally out of sorts, or you have troublesome symptoms such as pain or diarrhoea, your first thought is likely to be – what can I take to make it better? First aid for abdominal pain is a hot water bottle or the equivalent, and for diarrhoea there are several simple over-the-counter medicines which are worth trying:

- Codeine phosphate: 30 mg tablet three or four times a day.
- Diphenoxylate (Lomotil): two 2.5 mg tablets, three times a day.
- Loperamide (Imodium, Loperagen): 2 mg tablet three times a day.

None of these will be more than a stop-gap if you have Crohn's.

Steroids

The linchpin in the treatment of Crohn's is the use of steroid medicines – corticosteroids to be exact. Hydrocortisone is the steroid your body makes for itself, in the two small adrenal glands which lie next to the kidneys. As medicines we have a wide range of synthetic steroids, with *prednisolone* the most commonly used.

Back in the 1950s steroids were being tried – on the off chance – in several puzzling illnesses, ulcerative colitis among them. Since they proved helpful in that disorder it was an obvious step to try them in the other inflammatory bowel disorder – Crohn's. They have proved themselves the most effective and rapidly-acting drug treatment available, both in desperately serious situations or where there is chronic active disease grumbling along.

59

Severe, acute illness

In this situation, when your life is on the line, high doses of prednisolone can be injected straight into your veins. If your condition is not critical this treatment can be continued for up to five days, but then, if you are not much improved, it is time for the other option, surgery, to come to the rescue.

All steroids carry the risk of side-effects, and these may be dangerous if high doses of steroid are continued for long.

Moderately severe, acute illness

In this much more common situation, you are not desperately ill but you have several symptoms, such as a raised temperature, with loss of appetite, pain in the abdomen, diarrhoea – and perhaps one of the autoimmune reactions such as conjunctivitis or erythema nodosum (see pp. 41, 44).

You certainly need effective treatment. A reasonable regimen would be prednisolone, in 5 mg tablets: 20–60 mg daily in water, divided into four doses, for one to two weeks; then gradually cut down to 10–20 mg daily for four to six weeks, then taper off and stop.

Chronic active illness

Here the symptoms are mild, or die down only to return each time you stop the medication. To suppress the symptoms you will probably need to take prednisolone tablets for an indefinite period, in the following dosage: 10–15 mg daily at breakfast time, or 20–30 mg on alternate days, to lessen the risk of tiresome side-effects.

Risks

Steroids are wonderful in the way they relieve your symptoms immediately, but there is a price to pay. You must treat them with respect. Risky situations if you are starting on a steroid:

- If you have an infection, for instance influenza, tonsillitis, cystitis or TB, whether caused by a virus, bacteria or fungus. The steroid suppresses your body's normal reactions for dealing with the illness.
- Contact with anyone with chickenpox or shingles while you are on steroids and for three months afterwards. If you do get exposed to either of these illnesses, tell your doctor, as you will need immunoglo-bulin treatment at once and special monitoring. If you do develop chicken pox you will need specialist care.
- Recent operation or accidental injury.

- Recent peptic ulcer, even if it has healed.
- Diabetes, underactive thyroid, kidney or liver disorder.
- Osteoporosis.
- Glaucoma.
- Pregnancy or breast-feeding.
- Serious psychiatric illness.
- Stressful circumstances.

With children and the elderly you need to be especially aware of any new symptom or change and tell the doctor.

Interactions

You may already be taking some other medicines. Check that they will not clash with the steroid. Beware of interactions with:

- anti-epileptics
- blood pressure and heart medicines
- anti-inflammatories, for instance for arthritis
- rifampicin and other drugs for tuberculosis
- anti-fungals, for instance for thrush
- water tablets
- tablets used for diabetes
- erythromycin (an antibiotic), amphotericin
- salicylates, such as aspirin
- oestrogen, as in the contraceptive Pill and HRT
- anti-coagulants (they prevent clotting)

Main side-effects

- raised blood pressure, possibly leading to a heart attack
- water retention
- osteoporosis
- peptic ulcer
- moon face
- florid, red cheeks
- increased facial hair
- acne
- increased weight: fat body on thin legs – 'like a lemon on a toothpick'
- backache
- easy bruising, slow healing
- stretch marks on abdomen, bottom and thighs
- thinning of the skin

- muscle weakness
- impaired fertility
- depression or the opposite – euphoria with no cause
- in children, growth slowed down or halted

Dosage

Obviously, with all these unpleasant side-effects in the offing, it makes sense to try to cope with the smallest effective dose of steroid. It is preferable to take the dose in the morning, and on alternate days. It is safest to have a tiny regular dose (or none at all), and have a brief boost only when the illness becomes active. There is no evidence that a small continuous dose of steroid keeps you 'safe' during a remission; the on-off system is recommended.

Since the symptoms clear up so well with steroid medicine you may, naturally, feel that it is doing you good and curing the illness. Steroids have no effect on the course of the illness, but suppress your body's reactions to it, which comprise the symptoms.

Remember that you must not stop your steroid medication suddenly, but withdraw gradually over several weeks. Always carry a Steroid Treatment Card.

Topical steroids

Topical means that they are not taken into your bloodstream but are applied to the affected areas only. This means that the danger of side-effects is greatly reduced. Steroids are very effective locally, as is demonstrated in skin disorders, but with Crohn's disease the affected parts may be difficult to access, for instance, the small intestine.

Suppositories

Suppositories of steroid may be useful when the rectum is affected.

Enemas

Retention enemas are used in the treatment of Crohn's colitis, but the sensitive rectum may not let you hold the enema in long enough to do any good.

Foam enemas are easier to retain and feel pleasanter, but only reach into the rectum.

A special form of prednisolone is used for enemas (in France, betamethazone). However, if enemas are used very often too much of the steroid is absorbed and side-effects may kick in.

Infusions

Infusions or slow drips of steroid into the rectum are another method of treating the lower part of the intestines.

Poorly absorbed steroids

In the ordinary way steroid medicines taken by mouth are meant to be absorbed into the bloodstream as completely as possible, for maximum benefit. When a topical effect is required without a high risk of side-effects, such as for steroid enemas, a preparation which is not well absorbed but remains on the surface of the tissues is wanted. The most suitable steroids for this purpose include budesonide (Enterocort) and a special form of prednisolone.

Betamethazone, a favourite steroid in France, is very effective, but because it is well absorbed, tends to cause side-effects.

Reactions to steroids

Not everybody finds steroids helpful. You and your Crohn's may react to them in three ways:

1 Resistance – the symptoms show no improvement.
2 Dependency – you start off with a good response but the symptoms return as soon as you stop the steroid.
3 Prolonged response – the desired result, occurring in over half those who take steroid medicines for Crohn's. The symptoms are suppressed and do not return for at least a month after the steroid has been stopped.

The best results are seen in people with Crohn's affecting only the colon, or the colon and ileum rather than the ileum alone.

Emma

Emma was upset. These things matter when you are 23 and have a reputation as a head-turner. Something disastrous had happened to her face and her figure. Her cheeks were too red, and podgy – 'like a hamster', she said. And as for her figure! Her arms and legs were like sticks but her jeans and skirts simply would not do up: she had not got a waist. The doctor knew what it was at once.

A few months before, Emma had lost her appetite and a lot of weight – without trying – and had a permanent tummy-ache. Then the diarrhoea began and a funny rash came up on her legs. She was diagnosed as having Crohn's disease and started on prednisolone. It worked like a charm, but when she stopped it a few weeks later the symptoms bounced right back. Emma had been on with the steroid for another two months when she noticed these unwelcome changes in her appearance. They were the side-effects of the medication. The doctor reduced the dose gradually and then changed the prednisolone for sulphasalazine, a non-steroid. This kept her symptoms under control and her face and shape returned to normal.

Most of the other medicines used in Crohn's are aimed at replacing, if only temporarily, the powerful steroids and their side-effects, or at least enabling you to get by with a lower dose.

Salicylate group

Sulphasalazine

Sulphasalazine (Salazopyrin) and its modern relatives are the most frequently prescribed medicines in Crohn's disease. Sulphasalazine consists of two drugs: an anti-inflammatory related to aspirin, and an antibacterial, sulphapyridine. It was tailored for the treatment of rheumatoid arthritis, but turned out to be disappointing. The bonus for Dr Nana Swartz was that some of her patients who were also suffering from diarrhoea found their bowel symptoms improved considerably.

While it does not control the acute symptoms of Crohn's as swiftly and dramatically as a steroid, sulphasalazine is efficacious in mild to moderate exacerbations of the illness and for maintenance therapy in periods of quiescence. Applied directly to an inflamed area it is at least as effective as a steroid, so it is useful in rectal disease as an enema. Taken orally it is quickly absorbed, high up in the alimentary system, so there is hardly any left to treat the lining of the ileum.

Dosage

- 2–4 tablets (each 500 mg) four times a day during an attack
- 4 tablets a day for maintenance

Children over two years take scaled down doses, according to their weight. Sulphasalazine is supplied in tablets, suppositories, a lemon-flavoured suspension and as an enema.

Extra care

While there are no absolute contraindications, you and your doctor should be particularly alive to any new or unexplained symptoms if you are of retirement age, pregnant or breastfeeding, or have had kidney problems. Warning signs that the drug is not suitable for you include unexplained bleeding, spontaneous bruising, sore throat or general malaise. You need a blood test promptly to check that your blood is being made normally: a blood dyscrasia is a rare but dangerous reaction.

Interactions

Interactions may occur with other drugs: digoxin, folate, lactulose – make sure that you are not taking any of these.

Side-effects

- loss of appetite
- nausea
- headaches
- blood dyscrasia (see above)
- kidney problems
- hair loss
- pins and needles
- low sperm count

A third of those taking sulphasalazine suffer some side-effects.

Mesalazine (Pentasa)

This drug does not include the sulphapyridine component of sulphasalazine, so the side-effects are fewer, and it has no deleterious effect on the sperm count. It is particularly recommended for the other IBD, ulcerative colitis, but is less useful in Crohn's affecting only the small intestine. Nevertheless, it is replacing sulphasalazine as the most popular salicylate for treating Crohn's.

Olsalazine (Dipentum)

This medicine is not released in the small intestine, so it is useful only in Crohn's of the colon. Side-effects are uncommon apart from diarrhoea, which occurs in 6 per cent of users – when they may have this symptom already. A plus point is that not only is it harmless to sperm, it is also said to reverse any damage done previously by sulphasalazine.

Antibiotics

Metronidazole

Metronidazole (Flagyl) is another drug which was developed for a different illness and found to be useful in some cases of Crohn's. It is a first-line antibacterial agent for those organisms which thrive in the airless depths of the body, the *anaerobes*. There have always been suspicions that Crohn's is, after all, an infection, so it seems reasonable to try this particular medication. It certainly helps some people, but to replace the need for steroids it has to be taken in high doses, long term. This may lead to certain side-effects which are no problem in the drug's more familiar use in vaginal thrush.

Side-effects

- nausea, vomiting
- metallic taste in the mouth
- blackish, furred tongue
- pins and needles
- urticaria (nettlerash)

Very large doses, more than 800 mg daily, for a long period, can lead to a reduction in the number of white cells in the blood (leucopenia) – which reduces the resistance to infection – also epileptic fits, and possibly an increased risk of cancers, or of harm to an unborn baby. It is wise to take extra care with metronidazole if you are pregnant, breastfeeding, elderly or have had liver problems.

Interactions may occur with alcohol, lithium, some anti-epileptic drugs, and anti-clotting medicines.

Although there are many possible side-effects, metronidazole is often useful and usually harmless. It is more effective than clotrimazole or sulphasalazine in controlling the symptoms of Crohn's disease.

Immunosuppressives

In 1962 a Dr Bean introduced 6-mercaptopurine into the treatment of both Crohn's disease and ulcerative colitis, following the theory that since some autoimmune disorders occur with Crohn's (see pp. 43, 128), suppressing the immune reactions might have a beneficial effect on the disease itself. Dr Bean found his drug 'little short of miraculous', but then he disappeared into further research. In 1965 nitrogen mustard was tried out – effective but very toxic.

Azathioprine

Azathioprine, a close relative of Dr Bean's drug, was brought into use in Crohn's in 1966 – with success. In 50 per cent of cases it can replace steroids entirely and it allows a substantial reduction in steroid use in 23 per cent.

Side-effects

Azathioprine is very slow in building up an effect. You have to try it for four to six months to find out if it is the drug for you.

The danger period for one important side-effect is the first three weeks of starting the medicine, when, in the occasional person, it suppresses the blood-making factory in the bone marrow: a serious situation.

Other side-effects:

- severe nausea, fever, jaundice
- severe abdominal pain, sometimes with pancreatitis
- diarrhoea, which may be mistaken for a relapse of the original illness

Despite this unpleasant list, azathioprine is less toxic than steroids, and some patients have been taking it for as long as 18 years without side-effects. It is certainly worth a trial when Crohn's is complicated, extensive or resistant to steroids and other treatments.

Cyclosporin

Cyclosporin came into use for Crohn's in 1984. It is not absorbed in the small intestine in Crohn's and has to be given into a vein. It can be used in those who cannot tolerate or are resistant to steroids.

Side-effects

These include a a hot feeling in the skin, nausea and vomiting, tremor, overgrowth of the gums, and a tendency for the blood pressure to go up. Cyclosporin interacts with anti-inflammatories in common use.

Methotrexate

Methotrexate (Maxtrex) is effective in two-thirds of people with Crohn's, but it is toxic. It is used only in those who are chronically ill steroid failures, and those for whom azathioprine has also failed.

Side-effects

These include hair loss, infertility, a lung disorder called pneumonitis, upset to the digestive system and a low white cell count.

Interferon

Interferon is sometimes helpful in Crohn's and some other chronic disorders. It is given through an installation tube placed in the colon.

These last few drugs are used in Crohn's when the doctors are scraping the barrel. That is when the surgical option needs seriously considering.

Fish oil (MaxEPA)

Fats or oils are essential for normal life and growth. Fish oils are particularly rich in Omega-3, a type of polyunsaturated fat which is lacking in the lush Western diet. Omega-3 is even better than other polyunsaturates such as sunflower seed oil in protecting against high blood pressure and coronary disease. It is also an excellent anti-inflammatory, and worth a try in Crohn's. It comes in capsules.

Drugs still undergoing trials

These include the antileprosy drug, *rifabutin*, and two antimycobacterial antibiotics, *azithromycin* and *clarithromycin*. They all have numerous, unpleasant side-effects and until their efficacy is established, as well as their safety, they are not generally available (see Chapter 12).

Bernard

Bernard was unlucky. For starters he was 45 when he developed Crohn's, well past the regular age of risk, and then he had the unusual misfortune to be resistant to steroids. His main problem was diarrhoea. It interfered with every part of his life, but most particularly at work, where he had to keep leaving his desk. Besides, he was losing weight steadily and he felt weak. This was made worse by the anaemia: he was passing small amounts of blood on a regular basis, and his ileum was probably unable to absorb the iron he needed. Bernard had the common ileocolonic type of Crohn's, in which both the small and large intestines are involved.

It was a nuisance to find that Bernard did not respond to the steroids, but, as his doctor said, that left plenty of choice. Bernard did not mind what, so long as no one asked him to have an operation. He was not keen to have sulphasalazine because of possible damage to his fertility, so his doctor prescribed mesalazine (Pentasa). His symptoms began to settle, but some new ones appeared: he noticed big bruises on his legs when he could not recall any injury, then he had a sore throat. He mentioned it to his doctor, and a blood test showed dyscrasia with a low white cell count, so the medicine had to be stopped immediately.

Metronidazole, the next option, did nothing for Bernard's diarrhoea, but the doctor told him that azathioprine (Imuran), a more powerful drug, would be sure to solve his problems. He should expect to take it for two or three months before they could judge the effect. After enduring for several months a constant feeling of nausea and a horrible metallic taste in his mouth, Bernard was thankful to give up this medicine, too. Currently he is taking methotrexate (Maxtrex) and apart from losing most of his hair he has experienced only beneficial effects. The diarrhoea is down to three times a day, and Bernard hopes to come off all drugs in a few weeks.

Part 2: Surgery

It is something of a mystery still how most medicines work, especially in Crohn's disease. There is nothing to see, whereas with surgery there are instant results. Surgeons are straightforward men and women in the main. Their instinct is cut out what is diseased, and repair what is broken. The ongoing uncertainty about the root cause of Crohn's is frustrating for them, but there are situations in the illness which call for a surgical rescue package.

Emergencies

The chances are a hundred to one against your needing emergency surgery, but like a seat belt it is good to know that it is there for you at the crunch. Emergencies occur when one of the rarer complications of Crohn's arises.

Perforation

This is what happens when an ulcer or a fissure extends deeper and deeper into the wall of the intestine until it finally breaks right through, usually into the peritoneal cavity, the inside of the abdomen. There lie the closely-packed organs including stomach, intestines, bladder and womb. Perforation can affect either the small or large intestine, wherever there is a patch of Crohn's. Either way, it is a life-threatening situation, with peritonitis a practical certainty and septicaemia a grave threat.

The urgent surgical task is to stop the contents of the gut spilling out, cut away the affected section and divert temporarily the normal flow of part-processed food through that part.

Bleeding

Massive bleeding from an ulcerated area occurs most often in the large intestine, but it may have been made worse by a shortage of vitamin K, which is absorbed through the ileum – unless it is affected by Crohn's. This vitamin is necessary for the blood to clot. Apart from obtaining it from our food, ordinarily it is also manufactured in the large intestine by friendly bacteria. In Crohn's the bacteria are likely to be different, so this back-up production of vitamin K may not be available.

A major operation is required to remove the part, usually in the colon, which is susceptible to haemorrhage. A transfusion of plasma and a concentrate of blood platelets before the operation ensures that clotting can now take place safely. Ideally an angiogram – a map of the arteries in the area – is done before the operation, but this may not be feasible and time is of the essence. Bleeding from the small intestine calls for resection of the segment involved, but if the colon is affected total or near-total removal is the best option, with the provision of an ileostomy for waste disposal.

Treatment is essential for the anaemia which inevitably results from heavy blood loss (see p. 42). Leafy green vegetables supply vitamin K normally, and meat, wholemeal cereals and legumes provide iron. These are worth keeping to the fore in your diet, long term.

Toxic megacolon

This occurs in 20 per cent of people with Crohn's. It comprises the top emergency in sufferers and is a complication of toxic colitis, a serious condition in itself. An already extensively damaged colon becomes paralysed and swells up to enormous size, as much as 14 cm across or more. There is imminent danger of perforation, massive haemorrhage, abscess or septicaemia. In this situation *subtotal colectomy* (removal of most of the colon) is the safest treatment, and the sooner the safer.

Medical treatment, even if it holds the line temporarily, carries a more than 90 per cent risk of surgery being needed urgently, often in worse circumstances than if it had been done the first time round. Nowadays surgeons treat the healthy parts of the bowel very gently, in case they may become of use, and only remove the irrecoverably damaged parts. Antibiotics are used before the operation and afterwards.

Cancer

Cancer is a complication of very longstanding (ten years or more) disease of the small or large intestine. If it is in the ileum it tends to affect comparatively young men, but more often it involves the colon in older people of either sex. Regular check-ups, say twice a year, will catch the problem early. They must be thorough, and involve looking (endoscopy) and testing (biopsy).

If a cancer is found, prompt removal is the obvious course, probably with chemotherapy to follow. The outlook in cancer of the colon is particularly hopeful, much better than for other types.

Natalie

Natalie was 21 when she developed toxic megacolon. She had been in remission for several months and liked to tell herself that she had never really had Crohn's. She certainly did not tell Ned, her new boyfriend, about it. She was on the Pill, of course, and smoked about 20 a day. She drank moderately and liked to boast that she went out every night. To tell the truth, she had been feeling 'a bit off ' – in fact, ill – for a week or two when the acute, unremitting pain gripped her abdomen. It doubled her up and she went into shock. Her flatmate found her deadly pale and sweating. The doctor took one look at her, felt her rigidly hard abdominal muscles and dialled 999. He also rang the hospital. When Natalie arrived the preparations for surgery were already under way. She was given an injection of a wide-spectrum antibiotic almost immediately – no point in wasting time on a culture.

The incision for the operation, which would later be the scar, went straight down the midline of Natalie's abdomen, to give easy access to all areas. The diseased colon was removed and a new opening made, bringing the end of the ileum to the surface, an end-ileostomy (see Chapter 9). Natalie was whoozy for 24 hours after the operation, but well able to operate the automatic morphine injector on her wrist. After that she made a rapid recovery, to the amazement of her parents, since they understood it was an extensive operation. She said she felt weak but better in herself straightaway. She was no longer being poisoned by the toxic colon, the bacteria in the surrounding parts were well on the way to being wiped out, and a transfusion had topped up her own depleted blood. In fact, Natalie's main complaint was about the thick, hot, constricting anti-thrombosis stockings that encased her legs.

The ileostomy nurse, who had not had the chance of a discussion with Natalie before the operation, gave her a crash course in stoma care, and assuaged some of her horror and fear. All Natalie's friends, and they were many, rallied round and at times she was exhausted by their visits and phone calls. Ned was the most assiduous, and that made the effort to be sociable – whatever she felt like – worthwhile. Natalie has major adjustments to make in her life, but nothing, she says, that she cannot handle.

Elective surgery

Emergency surgery is forced upon you, as though a gun were held to your head. All other surgery is elective (Latin for chosen) and whether or not you have a particular operation, and exactly when, is up to you and your doctor. There is always an alternative, but choice is meaningless unless you have some idea of what is on offer. The bare bones are laid out below.

Elective operations

These are the likely reasons for them:

- Intractable symptoms – they simply will not get better despite the best medical treatments.
- Chronic obstruction due to a stricture – a narrow stretch in the intestine.
- Fistula – a passageway ulcerated through from the ileum or colon, into:
  - another piece of gut: *enteroenteric, enterocolic*
  - the vagina: *enterovaginal*
  - the bladder: *enterovesical*
- Abscess – a collection of pus, usually connected with a fistula.
- Chronic anaemia, from bleeding.
- In children, a failure to thrive, i.e., to grow properly and develop sexually.

Preoperative preparation

State of nutrition

This is always important in Crohn's, and vitally so before an operation. The success rate from surgery depends on being properly nourished beforehand. If necessary, as a boost to your nutrition and to give your intestines a rest, you may have a short period of *parenteral feeding*. A liquid is dripped into a vein like a blood transfusion, but containing all the nutrients your body needs. Such a 'rest period' for the digestive system used to be considered a treatment for Crohn's in itself, but it does not have a lasting effect, and it is too miserable to keep up for long. Two weeks on an elemental diet is another way of augmenting your strength (see Chapter 10).

Anaemia

Even if you have only been aware of having Crohn's for a few months, the chances are that you are anaemic. This needs correcting, and you will need iron tablets, folate tablets and B12 injections (see pp. 42–3).

Bowel preparation

The intestines are washed out (lavage) the day before the operation. If there is obstruction, or you cannot tolerate the lavage procedure, you have an enema two days running instead, with antibiotics.

Antibiotics

Unless there is evidence of sepsis or an abscess, antibiotics by mouth are sufficient. Otherwise they may be included in an enema or injected into a vein. Metronidazole and neomycin are those used in most cases.

Operations for Crohn's disease in particular sites

Stomach and duodenum

A peptic ulcer may also be present to confuse the issue, but the usual way for Crohn's in this area to come to notice is because of obstruction, due to the thickened inflamed lining membranes. The result is intractable vomiting. If the obstruction is in the exit area of the stomach and duodenum, the neatest solution is a *gastrojejunostomy*. The healthy part of the stomach is joined to the jejunum, the part of the small intestine that continues from the duodenum, thus by-passing the blockage.

If only the duodenum is affected, and the stomach lining is healthy, it may be possible to do a *stricturoplasty*, a kind of plastic surgery of the intestine which makes it wider, relieving the tight place without losing any tissue. This is well worthwhile, since with Crohn's of the duodenum, the ileum is almost invariably involved, too, and the less healthy mucous lining you lose from the digestive system the better in the long term. In rare cases the whole stomach may be so unhealthy with Crohn's that it is a relief to have a *gastrectomy*, removal of the stomach itself. This is not as bad as you might suppose, since so much of the digestion is done elsewhere, and a part of the intestine soon stretches to take the place of the stomach. Nevertheless you need a specially constructed diet and digestive supplements.

Small bowel

This is the area most typically involved in Crohn's, particularly the ileum. The usual operation is *ileal resection*, cutting out the diseased segments of ileum, often involving 25–30 cm of intestine, with resection of the caecum also. Some surgeons prefer a by-pass procedure, which preserves more tissue. The drawback here is that it leaves the diseased tissue to moulder, outside the mainstream of the alimentary tract. It is then slightly more likely to develop a cancer. The principle of trying to preserve all healthy tissue applies with either method. Once the area with active disease has gone, you are likely to shake off earlier feelings of lethargy, low spirits and malaise.

Fistulas

In these unwanted passages from one organ to another, so characteristic of Crohn's, there is usually the 'villain' of the piece, the diseased segment of intestine where the ulceration originated, and the 'victim' area which is healthy except just where the fistula comes through. This often occurs when Crohn's in the ileum is the source of a fistula into the healthy colon. In this situation only the fistula exit site need be cut out of the colon, plus, of course, the track of the fistula and the diseased segment of ileum.

Fistulas in particular areas

Ileosigmoid fistula

Nine times out of ten this starts in the ileum and emerges in the lower (sigmoid) part of the colon. Resection of the diseased part of the ileum is needed, but if the colon looks generally healthy only a small part round the fistula need be removed. The colon can be examined with a sigmoidoscope.

Rectovaginal fistula

An ulcerated passageway from Crohn's of the rectum tracking through to the vagina. The damaged parts need repairing and the motions temporarily diverted to allow healing to take place. The normal continuity of the colon is restored later.

Colovesical fistula

Running from colon to bladder, usually showing up through bladder infections and *pneumaturia* – gas or air in the urine (see p. 47). Removal of the section of colon from which the fistula arose and simple repair of the bladder puts matters to rights. While the bladder is healing, a catheter must remain in place for seven to ten days.

Fiona

Fiona had coped with Crohn's disease for five years, since she was 27. She was a methodical, rather fastidious person and had a healthy lifestyle with regular sessions at the gym and the pool, sensible eating and no cigarettes or alcohol. The only medication she took was an occasional paracetamol for tummy-ache, and codeine if her bowels were a little loose. It seemed most unfair that someone so careful and meticulous should get this unpleasant-smelling vaginal discharge and horrible pain when she passed a motion.

Even passing a finger as gently as possibly into her back passage or vagina was painful, so Fiona was given an injection of midazolam to take the edge off the sensations when an endosonograph was done (an echo picture). The course and position of a fistula from gut to vagina were examined and carefully mapped out, to help the surgeon.

74

Medical treatment with metronidazole and another antibiotic, a short course of steroids and a trial of azathioprine had all failed, so it was a matter of biting the bullet. Fiona knew she had Crohn's of the small intestine, but the source of the present trouble was in the rectum. She had to face removal of the rectum and the setting up of a colostomy.

The vagina healed well and Fiona's ambition, close to her heart, was perfectly possible, physically. She wanted to have a family. She mastered the management of her stoma, and acquired a degree of control over its functioning – but her sexual confidence was on the floor. That was until she had several months of psychotherapy. This rebuilt her self-esteem, and her partner responded to her new, positive attitude. Intercourse is now enjoyable again and Fiona is hopeful of conceiving. Her self-assurance helps at work, too.

Stricturoplasty

When there are skip areas scattered along the mucosal lining of the small intestine, a situation characteristic of Crohn's disease, the digestive and absorptive processes are upset. Carbohydrates are not taken in properly, peptic ulcers develop, vitamin B12 is poorly taken up and the colon is irritated by the arrival of inadequately digested fats. It reacts with diarrhoea. A low fat, high protein diet with no dairy products may help, with supplements of vitamin D and calcium, as well as injections of B12. Simple antidiarrhoeal medicines, such as Imodium (loperamide) or Lomotil (diphenoxylate) slow down the transit time of the material in the gut, allowing a longer period for digestion and absorption. Nevertheless, these manoeuvres have only a minimal effect, and weight loss is likely to continue.

More drastic action is needed, but resection of a long stretch of intestine – to include several separated areas of inflammation – would leave too little of the intestine to perform its vital work of enabling you to make use of your food. This is where the modern operation of stricturoplasty comes in. It relieves the narrowing, with its constant propensity to obstruct, without any loss of valuable, irreplaceable tissue. Several stricturoplasties can be done in the same session, which is useful when there are a large number of short strictures, separated by healthy intestine, or when several segments of the ileum have already been resected and there are no more that can be spared.

The operation is simple. A longitudinal incision is made over the narrow part of the gut, but it is sewn up horizontally, widening its shape. Complications are rare after stricturoplasty.

In extensive disease, a combination of stricturoplasty, as much as possible, and resection, as little as possible, may be the best solution.

TREATMENT

Crohn's colitis

Although Dr Crohn said it could not happen, it is no rarity for the colon alone to be affected by Crohn's disease. It can be recognized by similar features to those in disease of the small intestine – a variety of different types of ulcer, from superficial to very deep, skip areas, fistulas and involvement of the full thickness of the gut wall.

It is more common in males of all ages and seniors of either sex. There are three surgical possibilities:

- If an isolated patch of Crohn's is the only sign of disease in the colon, it is worth trying resection of that part only. It leaves you with a chance of normal bowel function, including passing your motions normally, for several years. Further surgery is usually necessary in the long run.
- If several segments are diseased, those parts only are removed, leaving the rectum and anus to work in the ordinary way (subtotal colectomy).
- Resection of the whole colon, including the last part of the alimentary system (proctocolectomy), often becomes necessary in the end. An ileostomy is constructed.

The first operation depends on the rectum and anus being virtually free of disease. In this case there is a 30 per cent chance of the desired outcome, with no need of further major treatment. In 35 per cent, the symptoms return after the operation, and the remaining lower part of the colon has to be resected and a colostomy or ileostomy made. Some people are so anxious to avoid this that they refuse the operation and struggle on with medicines, even when their symptoms are increasingly troublesome.

The big nuisance about Crohn's disease is that even if you have surgery, it is not likely to be the end of the matter. Crohn's can start up again anywhere. The recurrence rate of symptoms after all but one of the operations for Crohn's runs at about 50 per cent – but, on the other hand, you also have great powers of recovery. Proctocolectomy, removal of the whole large bowel including the anus and rectum, involves a risk of relapse of only 10 to 25 per cent.

Ano-rectal Crohn's disease

In this type there are, typically, deep fissures, fistulas or an abscess in the area, and passing a motion can be agonizingly painful. Suppositories help in mild cases, but surgery is usually needed. Surgery can relieve any constriction in the anus, while dilators may be useful to prevent its narrowing down again. Metronidazole (Flagyl) is definitely beneficial in Crohn's of this area and makes the surgery safer, but it is an adjunct not a

76

substitute for the operation. There is little evidence of metronidazole benefiting Crohn's in the ileum or upper colon.

Any child or teenager with unusual symptoms or appearances in the anal area needs a full diagnostic investigation to eliminate the possibility of sexual interference.

Crohn's disease of the appendix

Crohn's of the appendix only is a real rarity. The treatment is a standard appendectomy. More often the symptoms will suggest acute appendicitis and while the appendix may or may not be healthy, there is inflammation to be seen at the lower end of the ileum: *terminal ileitis*. If the colon is also involved it is called *ileocolitis*. Most surgeons would remove just the appendix if the tissues immediately surrounding it looked healthy, but would leave the appendix if there was a risk of making the Crohn's inflammation worse, and start medical treatment. In the rare situations where Crohn's of the end part of the ileum, the caecum and the appendix is causing obstruction, or the inflammation round the appendix is so severe that the tissues are breaking down, the only course is to cut out all the diseased area and make an ileostomy.

Relapse and recurrence

Most patients will need surgery at some stage in the course of their illness and there is an unlucky group who relapse regularly, so that they have to undergo repeated operations. They come to take the surgery in their stride, and malnutrition becomes their major problem. It is because of these people that the concept of minimal removal of tissue has caught on, replacing the old idea of taking it all away in the vain hope of getting rid of the disease once and for all. The game plan that evolved in the 1990s was to remove as little as possible. It had been shown that once Crohn's has been diagnosed it can appear spontaneously anywhere in the alimentary system, without direct spread from a diseased area.

Another disappointing factor is that no medicine, so far, has been found that reliably prevents recurrence. As with everything in Crohn's, a variety of different views and ideas are held. The good news is that the large pharmaceutical companies and surgical research departments are beavering away non-stop following leads to improve the situation.

Toxic colitis

Toxic colitis can be the first intimation of Crohn's disease, or a development in the course of a long illness. It is more serious than the more common Crohn's colitis, with a constant sword of Damocles threat

– the lethal complication, toxic megacolon. Even without the dangerous enlargement of the colon, an operation is regarded as urgent in most cases. The deciding factors are:

- Diarrhoea: more than six motions daily.
- Weight loss of more than 10 per cent of your previous weight.
- Abdominal pain.
- Pulse of more than 100 per minute.
- Temperature of more than 38.5°C.
- Distended abdomen.
- Colons looks big in X-ray.
- Laboratory tests show a high white cell count and low albumin (protein) in the blood.

Increasing distension, indicating the development of megacolon, is the signal for immediate action. The operation must be radical, involving one of the following:

- Proctocolectomy – resection of the whole colon to the anus, plus an end-ileostomy.
- Subtotal colectomy and end-ileostomy – by far the most frequent operation, and healing is usually trouble-free.

These used to be dangerous operations, but these days the situation has changed dramatically for the better. This is partly because the doctors are more likely to make the diagnosis earlier and start treatment, including surgery, sooner, while the dangers of toxic megacolon are widely recognized and looked for. In addition, sufferers today are more willing to accept operations as inevitable. Better antibiotics and more sophisticated aftercare mean that convalescence is shorter and patients are less liable to suffer setbacks. You can concentrate on 're-booting' your life, including especial care for your nourishment.

Richard
Richard was 33. As long as he could remember, he had been perfectly fit until, out of the blue, he began having non-stop abdominal pain, with eight or nine motions a day. He felt dehydrated but vomited if he drank anything, and his temperature hovered around 39.5°C. His flesh had fallen away, like taking off an overcoat, but he felt unaccountably happy and important. His doctor found that his heart was pounding away at 150 beats a minute. The clear advice was that he should go into a surgical ward for urgent surgery, but Richard was adamant that he would rather die than live with an ileostomy.

He was put on huge doses of steroids, antidiarrhoeals, antibiotics and immunosuppressives – but with no appreciable improvement. In fact, a new sinister symptom started up – Richard's abdomen began to swell, and his euphoria turned to delirium. It was only then, when his judgement was obviously impaired and his parents – next of kin – gave their permission for surgery, that Richard had the operation that saved his life. He had the standard subtotal colectomy and ileostomy, and his steroid dosage was gradually reduced.

It took Richard several months to recover fully, mentally as well as physically, but he did learn to cope with his stoma and get back to his career in computers, and the rock band that filled his leisure time. He tends to blame his parents for the whole affair.

This chapter has provided information about the basic medical and surgical treatments available in Crohn's. They may seem daunting, but there are the wide areas of lifestyle, attitudes, diet and your personal psychology which are also important. In these you have much more choice and control.

There is a mass of evidence that whatever else applies – infection, autoimmunity and other immunity problems, genetics – the environment has a major influence on the progress of the illness or otherwise. Why is it that Crohn's is so common in temperate climates such as North America and Northern Europe compared with hot, sunny Africa and Southern Europe? How do smoking, the contraceptive Pill, sugar and stress fit in? There is plenty still to be discovered, and meanwhile a great deal that you can do for yourself to keep well when you are in remission, and to help matters during an attack.

9

Ileostomy and colostomy

It is hard to take it in when you are told you are going to have an operation which means that instead of going to the loo in the ordinary way, your motions will come through an artificial opening in the front of your abdomen. The operation is either an ileostomy, which connects with the small intestine, or a colostomy, connecting with the colon. In either case the new exit is called a *stoma* (Greek for mouth). In the case of a colostomy it is usually below and to the left of the navel, while an ileostomy stoma is placed low down on the right.

You may feel that having a stoma is the end of the world, that you will be different from everybody else. In fact you are joining a club with 52,000 members in the UK (more than a million in the USA), with another 15,000 joining every year. The reason these figures don't seem to add up is because some colostomies, in particular, are only temporary. You won't know who the other members are unless you are close friends, but they can be anywhere, working in offices, selling in shops, practising any of the professions, swimming in the local pool . . .

Of course, you may still feel that you would prefer anything to having the operation – until you consider the alternative. Often a colostomy or ileostomy saves your life, and in all cases it will save a great deal of suffering.

Reasons for having an ileostomy or colostomy

Emergency situations

Perforation

When the Crohn's ulcerates right through the gut wall, spilling its contents into the abdomen, it will lead to a fatal peritonitis without an immediate operation.

Intestinal obstruction

This is another life-or-death situation. The first case record of a successful colostomy was in 1792. A baby was born without an anus – congenital obstruction. Death seemed inevitable until, on the third day, the desperate measure of making an opening into the colon was performed. The baby lived. If a narrowing or stricture of the small intestine becomes completely blocked, so that nothing can pass down the alimentary canal, it is urgent to provide another escape route for the waste. Nearly all those with classic Crohn's disease will need surgery sooner or later, because strictures are so common.

Massive haemorrhage from the colon

Heavy bleeding is not unusual in Crohn's affecting the colon – Crohn's colitis – and if you have lost four units of blood or more you need urgent surgery to prevent further loss.

Toxic colitis

This is a dangerous development in Crohn's colitis and it requires prompt action.

Toxic megacolon

This the top emergency – toxic colitis is a colon which has become huge and paralysed.

There is no question of delay in any of these conditions, but in others there may be time to discuss and prepare beforehand.

Non-emergency reasons for ostomy surgery

While some situations do not call for immediate action, an operation may still be necessary:

- To avoid unpleasant or hazardous complications, for example, bowel cancer. Long-standing Crohn's, especially if this amounts to ten years or more, increases the risk of small intestine cancer six-fold, compared with the norm, and nearly as much for colon cancer. Young men are the most susceptible to small intestine cancer and older people to colon cancer. It is foolhardy rather than brave to struggle on indefinitely with a melange of medication that is not controlling the illness satisfactorily.
- To put an end to chronic partial obstruction which is giving you increasingly frequent colicky abdominal pain, with the ever-present threat of complete blockage.
- Continuing failure to grow in children and adolescents: if nothing is done they will remain stunted and poorly equipped sexually.
- Longstanding sub-health, so that you hardly ever feel totally well – despite trying all the medicines, diets and alternative therapies.
- Physical complications such as fistula or abscess. A fistula (Latin for a tube) is a passage formed by ulceration from an affected part penetrating another organ, for instance the bladder, vagina or womb, or another section of gut. Chaos and infection are likely to ensue.

- Chronic anaemia, from persistent, maybe slight, bleeding from the back passage. The symptoms may include fatigue and shortness of breath (see pp. 43, 44).

You need have no fear that a knife-happy surgeon will persuade you into an operation you don't need, or remove more tissue than is absolutely necessary. The watchword for surgery in Crohn's is conservatism. Your doctors will want to preserve as much healthy tissue as possible, and only severely diseased parts of the intestine, which can never function usefully again, are resected (cut out). Of course, you will have the major hurdles of getting over the operation and of adjusting to new toilet arrangements, but the end result is that you will feel fitter in yourself than you have done for ages. With the removal of the diseased tissue, many of its ill-effects, both obvious and more subtle, are taken away too.

Ellie

Ellie had a difficult childhood. Her elderly father died when she was five and her mother ran through a series of men friends who turned out to be no good. The last one tried to seduce Ellie, who was then only 14, and it was in the following year that Ellie developed anorectal Crohn's disease. She had continual rectal discomfort, diarrhoea on and off and pain on passing a motion. Treatment with metronidazole, other antibiotics and various steroid ointments helped briefly, but the illness was getting inexorably worse.

A colostomy provided considerable relief. Ano-rectal Crohn's never goes into satisfactory, long-term remission with drug treatment. Without the disabling symptoms and reliance on a constantly changing regimen of ineffective medication, Ellie was able to live a near-normal teenage life. Music was the catalyst that enabled her to make friends on equal terms with her own generation. That was eight years ago. I have just received an invitation to her wedding to a violinist in a well-known orchestra. Something is going right for her.

Before the operation

Except in the direst emergencies, your surgeon will want to know as much as possible about the state of affairs inside your abdomen before he or she operates. Investigations are nothing to worry about. They may include:

- Barium enema – a liquid containing barium, which shows up on an X-ray, is given like an ordinary enema. It is vaguely uncomfortable but not painful, and takes less than half an hour. It outlines the inside of the colon.

- Ultrasound – not unpleasant at all, but you have to drink a lot of water beforehand so that your bladder lifts the other parts into the best position for viewing.
- CT (computerized tomography) scan, a comprehensive type of X-ray.
- Sigmoidoscopy – a flexible tube with a light at the end is passed into the back passage so that the operator has a direct view of the inside of the storage colon. The procedure takes 20 to 30 minutes but is no worse than uncomfortable.
- Colonoscopy – a fibreoptic instrument provides a view of the whole of the lining of the large intestine, and enables samples to be taken (biopsy) to examine under the microscope. You will be given a mild sedative during the colonoscopy, which takes about half an hour. It is the 'Rolls Royce' of investigations and provides the best and most detailed information (see Chapter 7).
- Ileocolonoscopy – a colonoscopy which includes the ileum.

After the operation

You will have already met your stoma-care nurse before the operation. Now you will be partners in getting to know your stoma and how best to keep it happy and functioning well. You will not be left to struggle on your own with this new, strange arrangement. Although it may be hard to believe, you *will* get used to it. It takes about three weeks to learn the essentials, three months to become expert enough to feel confident, and the rest of the year to complete your emotional adjustment.

Whether you have had an ileostomy or a colostomy, the essential equipment is a bag to collect the waste matter. With a colostomy this is like a soft motion. The material from an ileostomy, which has been less completely processed in the digestive system, is semi-liquid, like rather runny porridge. It is not possible to control this, but with a colostomy, you can acquire a useful degree of control over its action in three or four months. The equipment in either case may be one piece or two piece: either simply a disposable bag which fits over the stoma, or a base plate over the stoma, to which the disposable bag is clipped. Ileostomy bags may have a drain, so that you can empty them without removing them. For sport or some other activity you may want to have the bag completely empty although it is nothing like full.

The new toilet regime takes more time and more care than the old way, but soon slips into your daily routine. Diabetics are in a similar situation, but they have even more complex and fiddly health rituals – and really strict dietary constraints into the bargain. The many elderly people with incontinence problems also learn to cope with various appliances, and even the healthiest young women have periods to deal with.

Coming to terms and living a full life

Easy to say, but it takes character and persistence to win out against Crohn's, even with the support of those to whom you are precious and the professional help and encouragement you will receive. Your emotions have taken a hard knock and you are bound to feel both anxious and depressed at first.

Anxiety

Anxiety, sometimes peaking into panic, is natural and normal when you are faced with a new situation of having a stoma. Leakage is a big fear and the ultimate horror is that the bag will come adrift and you will get into a terrible mess. This is extremely unlikely because the appliances are made to fit well and the waterproof adhesive is extremely strong. Nevertheless, it is reassuring always to carry with you a set of spares, including underwear and a sponge bag: your insurance policy. All you need then, to set things to rights until you get home, is the nearest cloakroom.

Apart from this disaster scenario, which is not so terrible in the event, there are a number of lesser but more pervasive worries.

- *Other people will notice a smell.* No more likely than with anyone else. The most unpleasant, permeating human odour is that of sweat, feet and unwashed clothes. It does not apply to you.
- *The bulge of the bag is very obvious under your clothes.* Not unless you wear a skin-tight leotard. It is hardly noticeable even with a swimsuit, if it is patterned.
- *The stoma is repulsive.* It is normally healthy tissue, and no more unsightly than, for instance, the sexual organs, which everyone values so highly.
- *You cannot enjoy any normal pleasures, so you are cut off from your friends.* Not true. It takes a little more trouble, but you can swim, play sport, dance and have sex (see below). There is a mini-pouch to use during periods of physical activity and a sports belt to make things more secure.

84

If feelings of anxiety are interfering with your life, even when there is no special reason for them, it is worth learning some mind and muscle relaxation techniques from a psychologist or an occupational therapist. Ask your GP for a referral. There are also some audiocassettes which take you through the exercises. Breathing control exercises are also useful if you are liable to hyperventilate, while breathing in and out of a paper bag is a handy first aid manoeuvre.

Depression

As with anxiety, it would be unnatural if you did not feel a sense of loss and some sadness when you first have a stoma. The operation can come as a blow to your self-esteem – illogically, for you are still the same person, and worth just as much. There is a gamut of negative emotions which can grip you. Some people even feel guilty or ashamed – as though they are somehow at fault. Yet do you blame other people when they have an illness, or think less of them? Of course not. Nor will your friends.

Ordinary acquaintances will not know the situation and will judge you by the usual measures: kindness, cheerfulness, sense of humour – and most important of all, your interest in them. Of course you will get bouts of frustration and irritation plus a touch of anger of the 'why me' variety. You are not going to turn into a saint, so don't criticize yourself and don't try to be perfect.

If you are unable to argue yourself out of tiresome negative feelings and you feel low and hopeless most of the time, the life-not-worth-living syndrome, it is time to get help. This can be a talking cure with a counsellor or psychotherapist, but if you are losing sleep and weight, you need to see a psychiatrist who can give you antidepressant medication as well as, but not instead of, the verbal treatment.

Relationships, intimacy and sex

The single most consuming concern after the operation, when the life-and-death issues are out of the way, is sex. It has not usually been discussed in advance, so a man may be uninformed and fearful that he has lost his potency – as 55-year-old William put it, 'be only half a man'. While men fret about performance, women are afraid that having a stoma will be such a turn-off that no one could ever fancy them again.

For those who are married or in a stable relationship the fear is that their sex life will be in ruins, their partner can no longer love them and the marriage will collapse. In the majority of cases sexual habits continue much as before and the couple remain in the same relationship.

85

The physical effects of the operation are mild. A man may have a slight fall-off in his ability to maintain an erection, while a woman may find she can no longer achieve multiple orgasms. Much more important is the psychological effect. Sexual success is 90 per cent a matter of attitude and confidence. A follow-up of stoma patients in the 1970s found that after the operation:

- 85 per cent found intercourse easy, compared with 89 per cent before.
- 57 per cent had about the same interest in sex, 21 per cent had less and 22 per cent more.
- 75 per cent of the men could keep their erection satisfactorily, compared with 92 per cent before.
- 87 per cent of both sexes could achieve orgasm, compared with 90 per cent pre-operatively.

Not too bad a score, but psychotherapy is essential for those who cannot adjust sexually to the new arrangements. It usually takes around 12 months to recover from the operation and to adjust physically and psychologically. The partner also needs time to adjust, and joint therapy sessions can be useful. On a practical level, preparing for sex means emptying the bag and changing to a mini, or strapping it up out of the way, bathing and powdering, and covering the stoma area with adapted underwear.

Rita
Rita and Denby had been together for six years and had a little daughter aged three. Rita had struggled to cope with her Crohn's with fair success until she was 32, when she developed a fistula – an abnormal connection – between the small intestine and her womb. It made her life miserable and she was advised to have a resection of parts of the ileum and colon, with an ileostomy. Her relationship with Denby had often been stormy and sex was at its core. Denby found that he was now impotent with Rita – but not with other women. He would not go along with counselling, so Rita, a girl of spirit, said they should separate and booked herself in with a therapist.

She became increasingly independent, confident – and attractive – and after one abortive affair met a man who really appreciated her, made love to her and suggested marriage. Rita's little girl and Ed's young son have benefited too.

For the – so far – uncommitted, the problems are different. For ordinary social activities, your watchword must be *do* it – don't chicken out. The

86

tricky bit is when you meet someone with whom an intimate relationship is on the cards, with sex a looming possibility. The difficult decision is when to tell him or her about the stoma. Obviously, it is not the first thing you talk about with someone new, but it is a good idea to mention, early on, that you have had a major operation, and that it was for Crohn's disease. Crohn's has no unfavourable connotations.

Anyone whose feelings alter, when you come to tell them about the stoma, is obviously no use to you. For practical purposes it is no worse than having a part of your body under a bandage for some reason. Your sexual feelings are not doused by the physical change, nor is your fertility. Crohn's disease is no bar to pregnancy, and there are numerous cases of happy and successful mothers who conceived after an ostomy operation.

The crux is your emotional reaction. To ensure a successful adjustment, most people need a therapist since reassurance from someone who knows is a vital ingredient, as well as a sympathetic partner. Don't be fobbed off by anyone who expects you to be satisfied just to be alive. Life is for living and enjoying.

Embarrassing situations

There is no denying that you need a sense of humour when there is a stoma in your life. You are bound to run into some embarrassing situations.

- Your tummy gurgles loudly – grin and say it is the after-effect of an op.
- The bag gets full of gas and bulges, with the risk of making a smell – excuse yourself and release the gas in private.
- You are aware of a leakage – action stations. Get to a cloakroom and bring your emergency pack into play.
- Nosey-parkers try to bring the conversation round to how you cope with a stoma – don't be offended, be brief. Let it be understood that it is no more remarkable than any other private bodily function. No one wants to discuss how they clean their false teeth, either.

Eating and drinking

These can contribute to the embarrassing situations. There are no general dietary do's and don'ts for people with a stoma, it's a matter of finding out what suits you individually. This is a good time to take a preliminary peek at Chapter 10, Diet, and use it to check for details. There are a number of problems that are likely to crop up in connection with your stoma.

Wind, gas, flatus

We all have a certain amount, from babyhood onwards. Some of it we swallow and some is produced in the gut, from our food. It is embarrassing when it escapes through the stoma, or what is worse, gets trapped and causes discomfort and a bulge.

Swallowing air comes from smoking, gulping your food down, talking with your mouth full, putting more food in before it is empty, and drinking and eating at the same time. So – this is the time to give up smoking, if you ever did, avoid chewing gum, and eat with your mouth shut and not in huge chunks. Do chew your food thoroughly, so that it slides down easily. They say a ripe banana, mushed up in your mouth, is very helpful in preventing air-swallowing.

Food and drink that make wind include fizzy drinks and alcohol; beans, peas and sweetcorn; cabbage, cauliflower and spinach; mushrooms, turnips and nuts; and, for some people, milk.

Unpleasant smell

This applies to other people's motions, too. Watch out for the effects of asparagus, garlic, baked beans, the cabbage family, eggs and fish. You are more aware of any smell because both wind and motions come out at the front, just under your nose, under the new arrangements. As far as other people are concerned your fart is no more noticeable than anybody else's.

Loose or too frequent motions

These are often due to nervous tension. If you are feeling anxious, share the feeling and get it ironed out. Culprits on the dietary front are raw fruit, dried fruit, spinach, baked beans, chocolate and highly spiced dishes.

Constipation

If nothing is turning up in the bag or just a watery fluid which has percolated round harder faeces, you need to get your doctor's help and advice. You want to avoid a blockage, and it may be that some medication you are taking has a constipating effect, for example, iron pills or painkillers.

Odd-coloured motions

This is a not-to-worry phenomenon, unless the colour is due to blood. Nine times in ten it is caused by staining with a red food dye, such fruits as strawberries, blackberries or blueberries, or liquorice, iron pills or beetroot.

Remember that you are not a machine, and that your stoma is a part of you that, like other parts, may not always work perfectly. Teething problems may crop up in the first three months. Most of them are concerned with your learning the ropes, but the two important problems are obstruction and abscess. Since the stoma is so accessible, treatment is much easier than it would be if the trouble was hidden inside your abdomen.

Ian

Ian had been a life-long smoker – a 40-a-day man – and he had suffered from Crohn's disease since the age of 45. Now he was 67. Until this point, he had got by on a cocktail of pills and two localized operations for stricture. He had enjoyed some long periods of remission but these were getting shorter and his symptoms were troublesome. He was chronically anaemic and his weight was on the slide.

A new, keen, young registrar at the hospital decided to give Ian and his treatment regimen a complete overhaul, including colonoscopy and biopsy. Under the microscope the sample of tissue from Ian's colon showed dysplasia: a change from the normal structure. It was a warning of the likelihood of cancer developing. It did not mean panic stations, since on average there is a two to three year period of grace from the stage of pre-malignancy to cancer itself. The diseased colon was removed and a colostomy constructed. Ian's wife has been a tower of strength. She is glad to have him alive.

Some special situations

Travel

Always have your contingency supplies with you, and in your luggage pack twice as much of the stoma care materials as you could possibly need. It is also useful to locate the airport medical facilities, as a matter of routine. When Vivienne went to Rome, her baggage flew on to Jerusalem, but she had her emergency supplies to cover the situation until she could get to a doctor and a pharmacy. A *Travel Certificate*, rather like the orange badge for the disabled, can ease your way on the journey, for instance ensuring that you have no problems with access to a toilet. You may like to take a plastic sheet with you to protect the hotel bedding against any accident, but a towel is a lot more comfortable. Either precaution is likely to do more for your anxiety than to assuage a genuine problem.

Sport

Your stoma is as tough and resilient as any other healthy tissue. You do not need to feel that it is made of Dresden china. A sports belt to keep the bag in place will add to your sense of security, while for your swimsuit choose a bold pattern and the bulge will not notice. You do not need to worry that the water will cause the appliance to come loose. The special adhesive is stronger when it is wet.

Driving

Because your whole abdomen has been through a major procedure you should avoid the twisting and turning movements which arise when you are driving until it has had time to heal. Give it a month after your operation before you get behind the wheel again.

Work

It is essential for your psyche to get back to work as soon as it is sensible to do so. When that will be depends on the type of work. Heavy lifting is out for good. Because you have had major surgery, your body will be using its resources on repair and reconstruction. You cannot expect to have the energy, physical or mental, to manage a normal job, however sedentary, for three months. Even then it is wise to start by working part-time – shorter days or fewer of them. This will enable you to keep in touch with your colleagues and with what is going on.

Your prescription reads: sleep, rest, food and company. The last two are the most important – nourishment for your body and your mind. As for reading matter, a must is Dr Craig White's book *Living with a Stoma* (Sheldon 1997).

Because of my connection with the gastroenterology department, and my special interest in a group of brave people tackling the difficulties that can pop up in Crohn's disease, I cannot help knowing which of the people I see in and around the hospital have a stoma. There is that nice man at the library, for one, and the girl at the lingerie counter in Harpers; then there are the middle-aged couple who run the newsagents – she is the one with Crohn's – and, of course, our bank manager. There must be plenty of others I don't know about, living perfectly normal lives (with whatever effort it takes) – working, playing, laughing and loving.

10
Diet

Part 1: Diet in prevention and treatment

The key to coping successfully with Crohn's disease lies in how well you eat. To start with, you need to minimize the risk of developing the illness. Since good nutrition has been known for decades to be a protection against infection with mycobacterium tuberculosis, it is reasonable to expect it also applies to its cousin, mycobacterium paratuberculosis. This is particularly important if you have a relative with either form of IBD, ulcerative colitis or Crohn's disease.

Convenience, junk and fast foods

We know that people who make a habit of going for convenience foods – the polite term for junk – stand a bigger chance of contracting Crohn's disease. The special villains are white refined sugar and white refined flour, our universal Western addictions. Biscuits, cakes, doughnuts, pasta, pizza, pot noodles, white bread sandwiches and the bun round a burger – all are on the baddy list. They are so handy just to pick up and eat.

Sugar

The more complicated convenience foods, including savouries such as meat pies, baked beans, tomato soup, ham in packets and all the tinned baby meals, even bacon and egg, are laced with white sugar. The aim is to increase their palatability, since nowadays our tastes have been trained from babyhood to accept sweetness as standard. Natural flavours seem insipid.

Pure, white sugar can be used by your body as fuel for your brain and your muscles, and any surplus is stored as body fat, but it makes no contribution to building and repair work, which is necessary in ordinary health and even more so during an illness. It is standard procedure for your body to renew its various parts in a continuous cycle. For example, your red blood cells are replaced by new ones every six weeks, your skin is renewed every two or three weeks, and the lining of your intestines twice a week. Modern refined and processed foods have had the vital nourishment tidied away, removed from them.

Fats and oils

The other foods to beware of are certain kinds of fat, either saturated fats from animal sources, hydrogenated vegetable fats, or polyunsaturated fats which have been heated – for instance by cooking in sunflower seed oil. As a nation the British eat too much fat, especially the saturated type in dairy products and in or on meat, and this contributes to our high level of coronary heart disease and cancer, especially of the colon – which is related to long-term Crohn's disease. If you have Crohn's it is even more important to watch your fat intake. The damaged intestines cannot process fats efficiently, and this causes a train of problems. The exception is fish oil.

Additives

Junk food in general, with its artificial colourings, flavourings, and preservatives, increases the risk of Crohn's. The object of most of the additives is to improve the appearance and prolong the shelf-life of the product – not to increase its nutritive value. You must have noticed grapefruit and apples from far-flung places looking very attractive with a high polish. They have been waxed, to keep them looking good for longer. The downside is that the vitamins will have disappeared by the time you get to eat them.

Tarted up, processed foods, especially the fatty and sugary ones, are best avoided. If you like a cigarette with your meal try and drop that, too. It interferes with taste. You will find that after a short time you will begin to appreciate the subtler natural flavour of fruits, vegetables, wholemeal and other cereals, with protein foods – eggs, cheese, fish and meat – which have not been made into pies and sausages.

The only other item in general use which is known to make you very slightly more susceptible to Crohn's is the contraceptive Pill.

Food intolerance

One of the long-established theories about the causes of Crohn's disease is food intolerance, by analogy with coeliac disease. Certainly some people with Crohn's, but by no means all, find that particular foods make their symptoms worse. The lucky ones find that if they cut out these foods their illness goes into remission.

The food sensitivity or intolerance associated with Crohn's is not an allergy. Allergic reactions are usually obvious and immediate, and the tiniest quantity of the allergen – the substance responsible – is enough to set off the symptoms. Skin prick testing produces a reaction in allergy, but not in Crohn's food intolerance. In this a substantial amount of the specific food is required and the response comes on slowly. Since nutrition is of fundamental importance in Crohn's, it is worth exploring seriously which foods are good for you, and especially which you must avoid. There is no virtue in making yourself eat something your body rejects, either through the bowels or with abdominal pain.

You could be one of those whose Crohn's dies down as long as they keep to their personal restrictions. Some foods you would not miss if you never ate them again, but you are more likely to react to something you eat frequently. It is often the protein in the problem food that causes the trouble, but not invariably.

A long list of foodstuffs known to bring on symptoms in some people is given below. You will not be sensitive to all the possibles, but it is likely that if a particular food induces your symptoms, it will not be the only one. That is why it does not often work to try and find out if a specific food is the culprit simply by omitting it from your diet for a week or two. Even if you hit on one food that does not agree with you, the chances are that you will still be eating another one just as bad, and your symptoms will continue. To do the detective work effectively you need the determination and will-power to spend many weeks on an elimination diet – for which your doctor's supervision is essential. As a Crohn's sufferer it is not safe to disrupt an already precarious state of nutrition without expert monitoring.

The foodstuffs which head the list of suspects include wheat, dairy products, the brassica (cabbage) family, corn or maize, yeast, tomatoes, citrus fruit and eggs.

Milk and dairy products

One item that crops up frequently in Crohn's is sensitivity to *lactose*, or milk sugar, which is present in all milk products. The basic problem is a genetic shortage of *lactase*, the enzyme which processes this specific sugar so that the milk can be digested and absorbed. Lactase deficiency is not uncommon but Crohn's can point it up, and symptoms occur in reaction to milk in any form. It is particularly in evidence after an ileostomy. However, it is a mistake to deny yourself such valuable foods as milk, cheese and yoghurt, unless you are sure that doing so makes a substantial difference for the better. The most versatile substitute for milk is made from soya – most brands contain sugar to improve or disguise the taste, but you may be able to take sheep or goat's milk. Tofu is a soya cheese, and Quorn, from a fungus, is very much like a soft cheese.

Wheat

In this the trouble-maker is likely to be gluten. Fortunately there is a range of gluten-free wheat products available in health stores and the bigger pharmacies, but they are expensive. Rye bread, so long as it is

94

guaranteed 100 per cent, is cheaper and to be found in most supermarkets. Oatcakes, rice cakes and crackers, and rye crispbread can fill a niche.

Yeast

If it is this which is causing the trouble you can switch to soda bread, those large Scofa scones, pitta bread, chapatis, nan bread and matzos. The largest quantities of yeast are in Marmite, Vegemite, stock cubes, beer, lager, wine and cider and vitamin B tablets. You also need to be careful of pickles, dressings and cheeses, but spirits are usually tolerated well.

Brassicas

It is easy to avoid the cabbage family, and have your green vegetables as spinach, lettuce, and green peppers – plus those other vegetables, the legumes.

Tomatoes

Similarly, tomatoes can be side-stepped but may crop up in disguise in soups, pizzas and other made-up dishes. However, you may find that it is only raw tomatoes that cause trouble, and that you are able to eat cooked or canned ones.

Eggs

Look out for *lecithin* among the list of ingredients in manufactured foods. Otherwise, remember the egg in pancakes, waffles, quiche, Yorkshire pudding, egg noodles and pasta, brioches, cakes, mayonnaise, etc. There is no easy way of substituting for eggs and if you are a vegetarian, check that you are not depriving yourself of all sources of the B vitamins. These include wholemeal, green vegetables, Marmite, nuts and seeds – and for vitamin B12 you must have some food of animal origin.

Maize, corn

This comes as corn-on-the-cob, sweetcorn, polenta, and cornflour in soups, custards, gravy powder and sauces. It is also in cornflakes and some other breakfast cereals – so it was not such a crazy idea when someone suggested cornflakes were the cause of Crohn's disease (see p. 13).

Cold water has often been poured on the idea of food intolerance as an important cause of Crohn's disease – with some justification, since obviously it does not apply in all cases. Nevertheless, for some people it is the answer. May it not make the intestines susceptible to infection, perhaps by upsetting immunity arrangements? It was Dr John Hunter of Addenbrooke's Hospital in Cambridge who first took it seriously and carried out a series of scientifically planned, clinical trials, using a special, elemental diet.

Elemental diets

These diets contain no food – as we know it – nor micro-organisms. They are constructed from ordinary foods which have been broken down into their constituent chemicals, and then into the smallest and simplest molecules. Proteins, for example, are taken apart into aminoacids. The result is a liquid which tastes abominable.

Two elemental diets are manufactured: Vivonex, which is available only on prescription, and Elemental 028, which has been made slightly less unpleasant by the addition of a little sugar. As well as being extremely unpalatable, they are expensive, but if you have been diagnosed with Crohn's you may get them through the NHS. Since half the people who try drinking an elemental diet soon give up, the standard way of taking it is through the nose! A soft, flexible tube is slipped into one nostril, down the back of the throat and so to the stomach or duodenum. This way you do not smell it and it bypasses the taste buds. The tube does not feel as unpleasant as you might think. I found I barely noticed it after a few minutes, and you do not have to be in hospital to pour down measured doses of the 'diet' at the appropriate times.

The elemental diet is used in two ways: as the first stage in an elimination procedure, or as a treatment in itself. Either way, the point is that while you are taking this liquid you are not having any food which could trigger an attack or relapse of Crohn's. The absence of whole proteins is especially important.

Reasons for using an elemental diet
- in an acute attack, as one option
- as an adjunct to steroid treatment when progress is unsatisfactory
- undernutrition
- as a build-up before an operation
- pregnancy
- failure to grow in a child or adolescent
- in a young child

An elemental diet sounds dull and bleak, but it is nutritious. Delivered straight into the duodenum, it is full of calories ready to be absorbed.

After two to four weeks on the diet

- Remission of symptoms in 80 to 90 per cent of acute cases.
- Weight gain, particularly in Crohn's of the small intestine only, fairly effective if both large and small bowels are involved, but less so if only the colon is affected. Similarly, relapse is less likely after the diet if it is the upper reaches of the gut which are affected.
- Increased albumin in the blood, showing that protein loss is being corrected.
- Haemoglobin level rises, showing correction of anaemia.
- ESR lower, showing a reduction in inflammation.
- Intestinal permeability reduced.

(*Intestinal permeability*: If the gut lining is damaged by Crohn's disease, this allows bacteria to work their way deeply into the intestinal wall, causing deep ulcers, fissures and fistulas. One theory about Crohn's is that there is a basic genetic fault in the mucous lining of the small intestine especially – it is too permeable. Certainly the permeability is increased when the illness is in an active phase.)

One refinement which gives even better results with the diet is the inclusion of an antibiotic in the package. This is hedging the bets. Whether it is intolerance of certain foods or bacteria habitually living in the gut causing the symptoms, the diet-cum-drug treatment is bound to win.

Total parenteral nutrition (TPN)

Eight out of ten people with Crohn's go into remission on an elemental diet, and the results are similar with TPN, that is, when all the nourishment is given into a vein. It used to be thought that both these diets were effective because they gave the bowel a rest from the physical work of pushing the part-digested food along its length. Liquid food simply percolates down.

However, a carefully restricted diet which includes solids can be just as successful – it is not the mechanical rest which benefits the intestines and allows them to recover. Perhaps the absence of particular foods has an effect on the bacteria which live in the gut because *their* diet is altered. It seems that whatever else, the diets are more likely to be beneficial if the proteins in them are converted to aminoacids before they are eaten.

Mohammed

Mohammed had been brought up in Birmingham since he was three and had adopted the British lifestyle and eating habits. He also fell victim to Crohn's, the illness of Western culture, when he was in his twenties. He suffered badly. Because of recurrent blockage of his small intestine and an alarming loss of weight, Mohammed's specialist advised him to have a fairly limited, unhealthy section of his ileum removed. Nevertheless he was worried that Mohammed would not have the resilience, despite his youth, to recover quickly from the surgery. It was important to him not to miss, through illness, the revision course and the final examinations for his computer studies.

Two weeks on Elemental 028 had Mohammed ready to rebel against the regimen, but fitter and heavier than he had been for months. The operation went according to plan and Mohammed was able to sit his exam in June. He passed.

Although the symptoms subside – or remit – with the elemental diet they inevitably return, sooner rather than later, when the diet is stopped. No one could stay on it indefinitely. One answer is to have repeat periods of a few weeks, every time diarrhoea or abdominal pain starts up again. At one clinic the patients have four weeks' elemental diet every four months, to renew the beneficial effects. However, it seems even better if you can take a diet you can live with, long term, which avoids the substances your body objects to. The essential is to know which these are – and eliminate them.

Elimination diets

Dr Hunter found that more than three-quarters of his patients, who were all quite seriously ill in hospital to start with, recovered after two to four weeks on the elemental diet, and then reacted to specific foods when they were introduced on an elimination diet later. If they avoided these particular foods most of them remained well for the next two years.

Elimination diets are a ploy for detecting the offenders in food intolerance. They comprise three stages:

- Exclusion – all the foods you eat normally are withdrawn.
- Reintroduction – foods are introduced one at a time.
- Refurbished eating habits, omitting the trouble-makers.

The exclusion phase

The nub is that you cannot have any food that you normally eat. It is a test of will-power.

An elemental diet is a fine way to achieve this, and it rids you of your symptoms pro tem into the bargain. Some doctors give their patients five days on nothing but bottled water as an exclusion period. This is not a viable plan in Crohn's, because you definitely need all the nourishment you can manage. Besides, it is such an abnormal step that your whole metabolism is knocked topsy-turvy and this could upset your reactions in stage two.

If you do not need to go on an elemental, there are other exclusion diets, commonly used.

Pears-and-lamb diet

This or any other combination of an animal protein and a fruit or vegetable that you seldom eat. The point is to have something that your body has not dealt with often enough to develop a sensitivity.

Few foods diet

This provides you with a dozen rather than only two choices, but you must not pick your favourites. You must also miss out on:

- alcohol, coffee, tea including herb tea, and cola
- chocolate, sweets and candies, sugary foods and artificial sweeteners
- vinegar, pickles, highly spiced or salty foods
- take-aways, sausages, pâté, curry, smoked fish and ham
- restaurant meals

Your doctor or dietician can help you work out a selection that covers your body's needs. For example, you can have turnips instead of carrots, Quorn rather than cottage cheese, rye bread instead of wheat, etc.

Rare foods diet

One for the well-heeled foodie. It means hunting for the exotic, such delicacies as paw-paw, truffles, caviare, tapioca, pomegranates, pine nuts, chickpeas (a good source of protein), goose, rabbit, venison, pumpkins and pumpkin seeds.

A combination of rare and few foods diets is probably the most tolerable. The exclusion phase must run for three or four weeks, and it is a good time to get into the habit of noting down in a daily diary what you eat and when, your Crohn's or other symptoms, and your mood. This will be vital for stage two.

If you are no better after two weeks on your exclusion diet, the next step is to try a more rigorous version, even an elemental diet. Stay on that for a month. It will not harm you – in fact, quite the reverse. It supplies all your body's needs in the easiest form for it to take up. If you actually feel worse on whichever exclusion diet you had chosen, change to the elemental diet anyway – as treatment.

If you are improved but only slightly, it is probably worthwhile to stick with the diet you are on for the full month. There is no point in going on to stage two if you are not substantially better, but you have nothing healthwise to regret in having at least achieved the exclusion period.

The reintroduction phase

You may well feel deprived after the weeks on the exclusion phase, but physically and nutritionally you will be improved from the first fortnight onwards. You are into the positive part now. You and your digestive system will meet old friends, and sort out those that are not true friends but trouble-makers. It takes seven or eight weeks to work through the foods you have excluded, spending two or three days on each. Try each food two days running and watch for any unpleasant reaction – Crohn's type symptoms or headache, stomach ache, feeling sick or faint, vomiting. In this phase the diary of foods, symptoms and emotions comes into its own. It is a document you should keep for future reference.

If food intolerance is an important feature in your Crohn's, there will probably be two or three foods which your body rejects. If you react to five or more, this is likely to be a food allergy, unrelated to Crohn's and requiring specific anti-allergy treatment. When you have identified foodstuffs you must avoid, remember to look out for them in unexpected places – especially in cordon bleu type cookery, in which small amounts of numerous ingredients are melded together or concealed in a delicious sauce – enough to confuse any taste bud.

Refurbishment phase

This is the fun bit. You rebuild your diet along healthy lines, but scrupulously avoiding the bad-for-you elements. Aim towards the special Crohn's diet on p. 119, with the emphasis on high protein, low fat, plenty of fruit and vegetables and not too much of the very sweet. Foods you should include for sure (unless they are on your personal no-go list) are:

- wholemeal bread, potatoes, brown rice
- milk, butter (a little), simple cheeses
- cereals which have no added sugar such as Shredded Wheat, Weetabix, Puffed Wheat
- porridge
- fresh, unprocessed meat

- fish (not smoked), especially tuna and salmon
- beans and lentils
- unsweetened fruit juice
- lots of fresh fruit – raw, stewed or baked
- plenty of vegetables, especially green leafy ones and salads

Give your new, improved diet a month, then take stock, and adjust it as necessary within the guidelines. When you have carefully avoided a particular food for six months or more – I prefer a year – it is worth trying cautiously to find out whether your sensitivity to it has faded. Take small amounts only.

Rebecca

Rebecca was widowed at 43 and within the next three months her arthritis had developed. Fortunately the children, Paul and Beccy, were old enough to help when their mother's joints were particularly stiff and painful. The symptoms of Crohn's disease came on almost imperceptibly at the same time. To wake herself up and hopefully pep up her energy Rebecca had taken to drinking 'gallons' of coffee. She had probably sensitized herself to it, but just cutting that down had no appreciable effect. The doctor was worried about Rebecca's loss of weight – ten pounds in six weeks seemed too much to be accounted for by the bereavement.

The hospital check gave the answer: Crohn's disease. Drinking Hi-Cal and other nourishing supplements made very little difference to Rebecca's weight, and her abdominal pain and the diarrhoea continued. The doctor gave her a choice – to go on steroids or put up with an elemental diet as an introduction to an elimination study. She decided on the diet, encouraged by Paul and Beccy, and over the next few weeks she began to feel better, both in the Crohn's symptoms and the arthritis. She regained half a stone of the lost weight. The second phase of the elimination process showed that coffee and tomatoes were foods she must avoid.

She is now well into remission, including abatement of the arthritic pains. She is now a tea and fruit juice drinker. No tomatoes.

Part 2: Eating well

Eating well is an indispensable part of health, happy living, and for those of us with Crohn's it is doubly important. Unlike the tiresome 35 per cent of the populations of the UK and USA who are currently obsessed with shedding weight, you need every calorie you can get. It is not just quantity but quality your body requires. You cannot afford to burden your sensitive digestive system with rubbish foods and irritants, and you have a special need for vitamins and essential minerals. Although you are sure to be taking some supplements, it is wise to take the foods in which they occur naturally as well, for maximum absorption.

Why you should eat better than other people

1 A poor appetite – anorexia – is a common symptom of Crohn's disease. It is often one of the earliest and most pervasive. It means that there are periods when your intake is very small, so that what you eat must be especially nutritious.
2 An essential feature of Crohn's is damage, through inflammation, of the mucous lining of the digestive system. This interferes with both the digestion of your food and absorbing it.
3 The digestion of fats in the upper parts of the small intestine is often only half-completed and this has secondary adverse effects. Part-digested fat arriving in the ileum, lower down, cannot be absorbed but clogs up the delicate, specialized lining membrane. All absorption is further impaired. Pale, copious motions are a sign that too much fat is being passed out, undigested, with the waste.
4 Inflammation and ulceration of the ileum, the typical result of Crohn's, prevents it carrying out its function of absorption. This applies not only to the basic food elements – proteins, carbohydrates and fats – but crucially to the essential vitamins and minerals without which the rest of our food is worthless.
5 The digestion and absorption of starchy foods – that is, all the carbohydrates except sugar – is diminished because of the effect of Crohn's on the jejunum, which runs into the ileum. Carbohydrates comprise the bulk of our food.
6 If the colon is affected by Crohn's there is an extra loss of minerals. They are carried away dissolved in an excess of water which would normally have been salvaged by the absorptive part of the colon.
7 You may lose nourishment directly through vomiting, in an acute phase.
8 Diarrhoea means that part-digested foods are washed away down the loo.
9 While you have an active inflammatory process going on, including a degree of fever, you burn up your food faster.
10 Protein-losing enteropathy: when the intestines are healthy, they throw off a lot of protein with discarded cells, since they are

constantly renewing their lining. When they are irritated or inflamed this process is enormously increased and the small intestine in particular pours out water and valuable protein. You can easily drink water, but replacing protein depends on serious eating.

11 Post-operative states: if you have surgery to remove diseased segments of the small intestine you may be left with a restricted amount of absorptive mucous membrane. If you have an ileostomy or colostomy, especially the former, you will lose some of your fairly well-digested food, plus water, salt and other minerals. They literally go to waste.

12 Undernutrition itself, since it also starves the digestive system, impairs both digestion and absorption and it causes or increases diarrhoea. It can lead to a shortage of the trace metal, zinc.

13 Zinc deficiency reduces your intake because it makes food seem less attractive. There is a loss of the sense of smell, *hyposmia*, and of taste, *hypogeusia*.

14 Emotional disturbance: depression and anxiety are understandably common in Crohn's. Depression kills the appetite and anxiety disturbs the digestion, and by increasing muscle tension increases the demand for fuel.

Undernutrition

With all these reasons for an inadequate food intake, and an inability to make full use of it, it is no wonder that undernutrition is one of the cardinal symptoms of Crohn's. Some of its effects, apart from the vicious circle of the worsening of digestion and absorption, include:

- weight loss
- TATT – tired all the time
- low physical energy
- low mental energy, showing up as poor concentration and memory
- muscle weakness
- anaemia
- lack of protein
- feeling cold
- difficulty in shaking off colds, and slow healing of minor injuries

Other symptoms and signs might alert you to a deficiency of vitamins or minerals, in particular:

- mouth ulcers
- cracks in the skin by your nails and the corners of your mouth
- pale skin and membranes in your mouth or lower eyelid

- dry, parched skin
- bruises appearing with little or no cause
- ridges on your nails
- brittle, splitting nails
- sore tongue
- hair thinning

The effects of specific vitamin and mineral deficiencies are described in Chapter 3. If you have any of these signs and symptoms, see your doctor for a check – vitamins and minerals matter enormously to your health.

What to eat to provide the vitamins you need

Vitamin A

This comes in two forms: retinol, the vitamin itself, which is fat-soluble and comes from animal sources; and beta-carotene, a pro-vitamin which your body converts into the vitamin as needed. Overdosing on vitamin A is dangerous – Sir Ranulph Fiennes nearly killed himself by eating too much liver on a polar expedition, and there is a government health warning advising pregnant women against eating liver. The liver stores vitamin A. Beta-carotene comes from plants and carries no risks because it is water-soluble and the body passes out what it does not need through the urine.

Both vitamin A and beta-carotene are antioxidants (see below), and their advantages include a protective influence against some cancers and anti-infective properties for the skin and membranes.

Where to find beta-carotene

- carrots, dark green, leafy vegetables such as spinach and broccoli
- melons, apricots, pumpkins

These also supply fibre and vitamin C.

Where to find vitamin A

- liver (but do not overdo it)
- dairy produce, eggs
- salmon, sardines, tuna, fish oils

The vitamin itself is not destroyed by cooking, unlike beta-carotene.

Supplements

A special supplement of vitamin A is rarely necessary unless you have Crohn's, and only if they were unable to eat any vegetables or fruit would most people need beta-carotene capsules.

MaxEPA is a fish oil capsule: the eccentric spelling conveys that it contains *eicosapentanoeic acid* – EPA for simplicity – one of the essential fatty acids in the Omega-3 group. This has major anti-inflammatory powers and some research studies have reported remarkably good results in over half the cases of Crohn's disease. Instead of the capsules, you can take that well established stand-by, cod liver oil, or eat one or two meals a week which include oily fish – the flesh-eaters.

Vitamin D (calciferol)

Like vitamin A, this is oil- or fat-based, an antioxidant and not destroyed by cooking. It is needed for the absorption of calcium and zinc, but itself increases the demand for magnesium.

Where you find it
- oily fish (the carnivorous group): sardines, herring, mackerel, salmon, pilchards
- margarine (always has vitamins A and D added), eggs, liver

Sunlight on the skin enables us to make our own vitamin D, but dark-skinned people living in northern latitudes are at a disadvantage. The pale northern rays do not get through.

Supplements
Cod liver or other fish oil by spoon or capsule – see under vitamin A. In Crohn's you need to take a fish oil or eat oily fish regularly, but overdosage can occur. Take advice if you are pregnant or might be.

Vitamin E

This is also oily and occurs both in fish oils and plants. It is another antioxidant (see below). Because, with Crohn's, your digestive system may be inefficient in absorbing fats, you may require extra vitamin E. It is still controversial whether it has any useful role, but it has been suggested as helpful in a dozen disorders from infertility to diabetes.

Where you find it
- wheatgerm and other vegetable oils
- wholemeal bread and cereals
- butter and margarine
- eggs and broccoli

It does not stand up to heating or refrigeration.

Supplements

Capsules or tablets, including the chewable variety. The Department of Health suggests 3–4 mg as a suitable dose, but there are no agreed signs or symptoms of vitamin E deficiency.

Antioxidants

Antioxidants comprise a group of unrelated chemical substances which protect the tissues, to some extent, from the effects of *free radicals*. These are derivates of oxygen which hasten the damaging effects of ageing, degenerative diseases, and any chronic disorder. A sufficiency of antioxidants is especially desirable in Crohn's, and helps to prevent the development of cancer in later life. Vitamins A, C and E and beta-carotene are all important antioxidants.

Vitamin B1 (thiamin)

The whole complex of B vitamins is associated with digestion. Vitamin B1 is water-soluble which means that it is lost when vegetables or fruit are cooked in water. High temperature cooking like roasting, grilling, frying and also the canning process destroy it. Potatoes baked in their jackets lose their thiamin, but boiled in their skins they keep most of it. Preservatives and baking powder destroy it, and even chopping, mincing or liquidizing the food means the loss of three-quarters of the vitamin.

Where to find it

- Luckily that staple food, wholemeal bread, is an excellent source – so long as you do not toast it.
- Other whole-grain cereals, wheatgerm, pasta, rice and yeast.
- Kidneys, liver and pork.

There is no risk from accidental overdose, since any surplus is disposed of in the urine, but it reacts with *levodopa*, a medicine for Parkinson's disease. You can run short of thiamin because of poor absorption from the small intestine, or if you drink alcohol in excess. It is worth ensuring an adequate supply because it appears to have a beneficial effect on the intestines, since it speeds up recovery from gastroenteritis.

Supplements

A daily compound vitamin B tablet will supply all you need.

Vitamin B2 (riboflavin)

This vitamin contributes to the digestion and efficient usage of both carbohydrates and proteins, and it facilitates the absorption of iron, vitamin B6 and folate. It stands up quite well to cooking, but deteriorates if exposed to sunlight – the milk bottle left on the doorstep all day. This does not matter to most people, because it abounds in a wide variety of foods, but with Crohn's you need to make sure that you have enough of so important a vitamin.

Where to find it
- milk and cheese (the main sources)
- liver, kidney, Marmite, eggs, wheatgerm and bran, cereals with commercially added vitamins

Supplement

A daily B-complex tablet is likely to be sufficient. The minimum dose is 1 mg daily, but you will require 3–4 mg, plus extra if you are taking a tricyclic antidepressant, such as amitriptyline, or the tranquillizer, chlorpromazine. Overdosage is not a danger.

Lack of riboflavin is reputed to be the cause of cracks in the corners of the mouth and a sore, red tongue, but other conditions, for instance a shortage of niacin, vitamin C or iron may be responsible.

Vitamin B3 (niacin, nicotinic acid)

This stimulates your circulation and helps with chilblains and painful periods. It also makes your skin feel hot. You must not take it in tablet form if you have a peptic ulcer.

Where you find it
- yeast, Marmite, peanuts, bran
- wholemeal, coffee
- liver, kidney, meat, fish

Supplement

Again, the B-complex tablet will include enough niacin.

Vitamin B6 (pyridoxine)

B6 is necessary for amino-acid metabolism, enabling you to make best use of your proteins – something you are likely to lack. It also has a beneficial effect on mood, especially the depression sometimes associated with taking oestrogens – the Pill or HRT.

Where you find it
- liver, kidneys, meat, fish, eggs
- whole grain cereals, potatoes
- bananas, avocados, walnuts, Royal jelly

It will survive gentle cooking.

107

Vitamin B12 (cobalamin)

This was not isolated until 1948. Before that people like George Bernard Shaw, who suffered from a serious form of anaemia, had to eat large quantities of liver. Now cobalamin can be given by injection. The related anaemia that arises in Crohn's is due to the failure of the small intestine to absorb this vitamin and its partner, folic acid. There is a very high risk of B12 supplies falling short after surgery to remove diseased parts of the ileum. The treatment of this anaemia is the same as in GBS's pernicious type: regular three-monthly injections.

Where you find it
• liver, kidney, sardines, oysters, meat
• eggs, cheese, milk

Because it is found in animal sources only, vegans are highly susceptible to a dangerous B12 deficiency, with physical and mental symptoms. A diet that excludes meat is unsafe in Crohn's (see Chapter 3).

Folic acid, folates

This vitamin gets its name from *foliage*, the leaves of a plant, because that is where you find it. It works in collaboration with vitamin B12 in the manufacturing and maturing of red blood corpuscles in the bone marrow. The two are also involved in the production of DNA, the blueprint chemical for your whole body. A lack of folate brings on all the anaemic and other symptoms of B12 deficiency. Folic acid is particularly important in pregnancy.

Where you find it
• green, leafy vegetables, lettuce and beetroot
• oranges, bananas and avocados
• wholemeal bread, bran, eggs and uncooked peanuts

Supplement
A daily tablet ensures an adequate supply. There is no overdosage problem.

Vitamin C (ascorbic acid)

This is another antioxidant, hopefully protecting the tissues, including those of the digestive system, from succumbing too fast to wear and tear. Injuries and Crohn's ulcers heal better with plenty of vitamin C, and in the treatment of anaemia it helps the absorption of iron. Plenty does not mean mega-doses, however, since they can lead to withdrawal symptoms.

We do not see scurvy these days, but a shortage of vitamin C shows itself by spontaneous bruising, anaemia and spongy, friable gums. People in hospital, or other institutions where there is mass catering, are often short of vitamin C: it has been cooked away, and fresh foods tend to be a rarity in such places.

Where you find it

- blackcurrants (including blackcurrant drinks), citrus fruits, guavas
- green peppers, salad vegetables (raw)
- vegetables of the brassica group: cabbage, broccoli, sprouts, cauli-flower – as crudités or lightly cooked
- potatoes, milk

It is quickly destroyed by cooking, exposure to the air, and by cutting, peeling and washing.

Supplement

Since your body can neither make this vitamin nor store it, it is sensible to make sure of your daily intake, in winter especially, by taking a daily tablet. Even if you are not anaemic – but more so if you are – vitamin C gives a boost to your feeling of energy.

Unfortunately several medicines work against vitamin C, including steroids, which are very relevant to Crohn's; also aspirin, tetracycline and indomethacin.

Vitamin K

The 'K' comes from the word for coagulation in Danish, because this vitamin is necessary for the blood to clot. It comes in two forms: K1 and K2. K1 can be lacking in Crohn's through poor absorption, and K2 because of a change of bacteria in the colon in the illness.

Where you find it

- green, leafy vegetables like spinach
- cauliflower
- lucerne (alfalfa)
- manufactured in the colon by some friendly strains of E. coli

Supplement

If a clotting time test shows that you are low in vitamin K, which could lead to severe bleeding from ulcerated areas, tablets or injections are available.

Minerals

Some chemicals play an important role in the structure and functioning of
your body – think of iron in your blood and calcium in your bones. Only
very small amounts are required, but they are absolutely vital. With
Crohn's you are in a vulnerable situation because of the double whammy
of poor absorption and extra losses through the bowels.

Calcium

This is important for the health and strength of bones and teeth,
especially in children and the elderly. Children with Crohn's are in
danger of poor, stunted growth, particularly affecting the long bones –
adequate supplies of calcium are vital. Pregnant women need extra
supplies and from middle age onwards there is the spectre of osteoporosis. Calcium is also concerned in the nerves supplying the muscles.
Everyone needs vitamin D to be able to absorb calcium, especially the
vulnerable groups including people with Crohn's or anorexia nervosa.

Where you find it
- cheese, milk, yogurt
- fish eaten with the bones: sardines, pilchards, whitebait
- peanuts, almonds, chickpeas, beans
- eggs, bread to which calcium has been added (see *Phytates*, below)

Iron

Iron is an essential ingredient of haemoglobin, the oxygen-carrying
compound in red blood cells. It is so precious that it is salvaged and
recycled by the body – but in Crohn's it is poorly absorbed and often lost
in the motions in diarrhoea. Iron deficiency anaemia is so common as to
be almost standard in Crohn's (see p. 42).

Where you find it
- meat, poultry, liver, fish (especially sardines), eggs
- wholemeal cereals, oatmeal, All-bran (see *Phytates*, below)
- peas, beans, lentils, spinach
- prunes, raisins
- chocolate

Vitamin C enhances the absorption of iron, but tea and coffee inhibit it.
Vegetarians, even without Crohn's, often become iron-deficient, and

should never drink tea or coffee with their meal. If you are a Crohn's sufferer it is vital not to restrict your diet.

Supplement

You probably need to take iron tablets anyway, but for sure if you have either type of anaemia. In some people they cause pain and disturbance of the intestines, either constipation or diarrhoea, but there are several different preparations, one of which might suit you.

Magnesium

This is necessary for the health of the brain and nerves. A lack of it can cause depression, agitation or confusion. You can run short of magnesium in Crohn's because of general undernutrition, diarrhoea or vomiting.

Where to find it

- cocoa, plain chocolate
- cashews, almonds, brazil nuts
- shrimps and prawns
- barley, wheat, peas and beans

Supplement

You can buy tablets in health food shops, but it is better to take it in your diet. (See *Phytates*, below.)

Zinc

Zinc deficiency was first recognized in 1972, and it is now established that the absence of the tiny amount that is all the body needs can cause far-reaching effects. They include diarrhoea, mental apathy, weakness of the muscles, nerve pain, and a loss of the senses of smell and taste.

Where you find it

- oysters – or for most of us, sardines
- meat and liver
- wholemeal, oatmeal, breakfast cereals
- nuts, peas and beans

Supplement

Zinc can run short in Crohn's from malabsorption and losses in the motions. Tablets may be used to ensure an intake of 15 mg a day. (See *Phytates*, below.)

Selenium

This is another antioxidant and can be beneficial in Crohn's. Its action is related to that of vitamin E, but little else is known about it.

Where to find it

- Wholemeal bread and other wholemeal foods, especially if they come from grain grown in America (European soil contains very little selenium).
- Brazil nuts.

Supplement

Tablets are available in health stores, but there is little reason to suppose it will benefit you.

Phytic acid, phytates

If you pride yourself on a healthy diet, never eating white bread or sugared cornflakes, but wholemeal everything from scones to chapattis, oats for breakfast as porridge or muesli, and bran scattered ad lib, you will be in fashion. You may also be depriving your body of some essential minerals. Simply using plenty of bran – because 'it is good for you' – can cause serious mineral deficiencies, because of the phytates in it.

They do their damage by latching on to iron, calcium, zinc and magnesium and forming insoluble compounds which cannot be absorbed, and are passed out with the motions. Fortunately wholemeal *bread* retains its iron and calcium in particular, because the yeast in it counteracts the phytate. And you can make a (health) case for eating phytate-free white bread whenever you fancy a change.

Fibre

This is a food which provides us with no nourishment, yet it is necessary to our health, especially the small and large intestines. Its value was first brought to notice by an Englishman, Dr T. R. Allinson, and two Americans, Dr John Harvey Kellogg and the philanthropist Sylvester Graham. Graham's crackers are a kind of digestive biscuit.

An earlier term was *roughage*, then came *fibre*, and since the early 1990s the Department of Health has said:

- We should have more of it.
- We should call it *non-starch polysaccharides* – NSP for short.

I prefer the term fibre. In essence it comprises all the parts of a plant that we cannot digest. There are several different sorts, for example, pectin, cellulose, hemicellulose and lignin. They are all carbohydrates. Their most remarkable feature is their ability to absorb water – 15 times their own weight. This makes for a motion that is firm but soft, and causes no irritation as it passes down the gut. It also increases the bulk of the motion.

Fibre is particularly beneficial in Crohn's, when poor appetite and impaired functioning of the gut may produce a motion that is too little and too liquid to stimulate movement or to control.

Our current preference for highly refined, processed foods – white bread, cakes and buns, polished rice, and sugar as pure, white sucrose – deprive the small and large intestines of the exercise they need to keep fit. A low fibre diet can lead to constipation in the short term, but more seriously and insidiously, over time, to diverticular disease, gallstones, irritable colon and ultimately colon cancer.

The recommended intake should be between 12 and 32 grams daily (32 g is a little over an ounce – it weighs light).

Where to find it
- bran, bran cereals like All-bran
- wholemeal, oatmeal, brown rice
- dried fruit, especially prunes
- potatoes in their jackets, especially the jackets
- raw, fresh fruit, especially bananas
- salads, green vegetables, nuts

By far the best source is bran, either wheat or oat. The latter is preferable because it contains less phytate. This means that not as much of the minerals iron, calcium, zinc and magnesium is made unabsorbable (see *Phytates*, above). A test of whether you are taking enough fibre is to check whether your motion sinks like a stone in the loo, or tends to float. Fibre is light.

Some high-fibre foods may cause gas indigestion. An excess of gas is produced in the colon, causing pain and bloating. Taking iron pills – usually for anaemia – sometimes alleviates the situation.

Your immune system

Since your immune system is your main defence force against the enemies of your body, including any sneaky bugs that are involved in Crohn's disease, it is essential to supply it with the fuel it needs.

The organization of the immune system

The immune system accounts for 2 per cent of your body weight – the same amount as your brain. It consists of cells produced in the bone marrow, some of which travel all over your body – a mobile fighting force – while others aggregate together in lymph glands. Some are dispersed between other cells in the lining of intestine.

The immune cells come in two major families, the Ts and the Bs.

The T cells

- *T helper cells* assess the dangers and switch on the immune system when necessary. These cells are knocked out by the AIDS virus.
- *T suppressor cells* switch the system off when the attack is over.
- *T cytotoxic cells* are killers – of cancer cells and other undesirables.
- *T DTH cells* mediate delayed hypersensitivity, which may be relevant to reactions to food or bacteria in Crohn's disease.

T cells are able to cope with bacteria, fungi and viruses that get inside healthy cells.

The B lymphocytes

These cells make up the mobile fighting force which homes in on trouble spots, such as patches of Crohn's, an injury or an infection. There are several types.

- *Polymorphonuclear granulocytes* (polymorphs for short): they kill and eat invaders. You are a pushover for infections if you run short of these.
- *Macrophages*: polymorphs are small but macrophages are large (macro = big), and they also swallow up germs of all types and also cancer cells. They lurk around in the vicinity of an infection, inflammation or tumour. As well as attacking baddies, they trigger local blood clotting, and are instrumental in the repair and remodelling of damaged tissues.
- *NK (natural killer) cells*: their special mission is to root out viruses and destroy them.

The B cells produce antibodies, chemical substances called immunoglobulins. These come in different classes – IgG is the commonest. They deal with specific enemies. For instance they immobilize the diphtheria germ so that a polymorph or macrophage can gobble it up. IgA (Immunoglobulin A) is a special for gut problems. It confers a measure of immunity to unfriendly bacteria and can sort out the good from the bad.

114

What the immune system needs

Minerals

- *Calcium* is needed by the macrophages and polymorphs in particular, and works in conjunction with magnesium. Root vegetables are the best source of magnesium.
- *Iron* boosts overall resistance to infection. Too much in concentrated form can be toxic so try and get all you can through your food, helped by vitamin C.
- *Zinc and selenium* are both useful antioxidants. Zinc is needed in the maturation of T cells and selenium in antibody production.

Vitamins

- *Vitamin A* is particularly effective where there is a high risk of infection, such as the nose and throat, the genital and urinary areas and, of course, the bowels. It is used in the production of lysozyme, an antibacterial enzyme found in tears, sweat and saliva and other body fluids.
- *B complex vitamins*, especially B12 and folic acid, are involved in all types of healing, including that of Crohn's ulcers, and of growth in the young. B6, pyridoxine, is used by the cells which eat up invaders.
- *Vitamin C* slows down the rate of multiplication of most viruses, and boosts the production of both T and B leucocytes.

Immune system suppressors

Obviously, after an infection or other attack on the body has passed or healed, you do not need the immune system working at full blast. It would be like having the central heating full on in midsummer. The T suppressor cells switch it off as needed, but some other substances and some circumstances suppress the immune system just when you need it. They include:

- Vitamin D in excess.
- Coffee, tea and other stimulants (Speed, cocaine, Ecstasy).
- Alcohol and cannabis. Both of these stimulate briefly, then suppress the immune system. This mirrors the psychological effect of drinking – you are happy and witty after the first glass but as you take more you function less efficiently.
- Missing a whole night's sleep (alternately drowsing and waking all night does not count).

- Chronic stress, leading to irritability and pessimism.
- Lack of fresh air, exercise, or social contacts.
- Lack of an intimate relationship, including sex.
- Breathing polluted air – exhausting for your immune system.

Part 3: Constructing your personal diet

What will serve you and your body best will vary with the state of your Crohn's disease and your personal situation at the time.

- Is the illness active, recovering or in remission?
- Have you a stoma to consider, after an ostomy?
- Are you pregnant?
- Are you still growing?
- Are you under any particular strain?

The mix of nourishment most likely to keep you well during remission, or to aim towards after a rough patch, includes many of the elements of an anti-cancer diet. The foundation stones are proteins, carbohydrates and fats, and in Crohn's you need all the trimmings – vitamins and minerals, and fibre. You need more calories than other people, so do not hold back, on proteins especially, and also carbohydrates, but go canny with fats and highly refined sugar.

First and most important – you must enjoy your meals. A poor appetite is one of the bugbears of Crohn's. Any special cause needs putting right but there are some general guidelines.

- Aim for pleasant surroundings and pleasant company, and when you are at home make your table or tray look attractive – for you.
- Allow plenty of time to eat, and slow the pace by reading a book if you are on your own. It helps your digestive system if you chew each mouthful properly and enables you to appreciate flavours to the full.
- Choose simple foods, but of the top quality. It is false economy to fob your body off with second best, when food is fundamental to your health.

Special circumstances

Pregnancy

If your Crohn's is quiescent all you need to do is avoid liver, lightly cooked eggs and cheeses other than cottage cheese or cheddar, and to make very sure of having foods which contain all the vitamins and essential minerals. Folate is especially important and you need a supplement, probably a multivitamin and mineral type. Babies are built on protein, so make sure you have your daily quota.

If your Crohn's is playing up, a formula diet, including an elemental, is safe and particularly effective in pregnancy.

Children and adolescents

Young children who are not growing at a satisfactory rate may need to have a course of tube feeding to get the extra nutrition on board. An adolescent who is lagging behind in height or sexual development also urgently requires a boost. An elemental or less severe formula diet, by tube if necessary, will save him or her from permanently stunted growth and reproductive immaturity. Calcium with vitamin D is needed for growing bones, and again – plenty of protein. This is not the time to turn vegetarian, since it is difficult to eat enough of the pulses and grains to supply vegetarian protein – apart from the need for vitamin B12, from animal sources.

With an ileostomy or colostomy

After these operations the colon will no longer be available to reabsorb water and the essential minerals dissolved in it. Normally it absorbs a litre of water a day. With an ileostomy it is not only the scarce minerals such as iron and magnesium that need replacing, but after an ileostomy you also lose a great deal of salt (sodium chloride). Both fluid and minerals, especially salt, must be made up, and supplements are necessary. Ileostomy diarrhoea is a common complication which serves to intensify the problem.

The giant strides in how you feel a few months after an ostomy are well worth a few adjustments in your intake.

Diarrhoea

It is likely that from time to time this symptom will crop up, or it may be a long-term tendency in your case. In the acute stage you may be restricted to plenty of such drinks as lemon barley water or very weak tea, with dry toast or Marie biscuits. In the recovery phase, or if you are often liable to diarrhoea, go for:

- small, frequent meals
- smooth, unstimulating food without condiments, spices or pickles
- nothing very hot or refrigerated
- plenty to drink, especially betwen meals
- enough protein, B-complex vitamins and vitamin C

Don't have:

- alcohol, strong tea or coffee
- meat extracts
- fried food
- fresh bread or hot buttered toast
- sausages, bacon, pork, twice-cooked meat; visible fat on meat
- unripe or dried fruit

Bland diet

A diet for when you are recovering from an attack and need to build up gently.

On waking	Weak tea with milk and sugar Marie or Rich tea biscuit
Breakfast	Strained porridge or Weetabix, with milk and pureed fruit Egg or tiny portion of steamed white fish Crisp toast, spread when cold Runny honey, jelly marmalade, or golden syrup
Mid-morning	Milky drink, banana or biscuit
Lunch	Fish, lean, tender meat or chicken, or soft cheese Sieved vegetables, e.g. broccoli and carrots, plus mashed potatoes, pasta or crisp toast Yogurt, fromage frais or rice pudding with sieved fruit, or fruit fool or jelly, or stewed or baked apple Diluted fruit drink
Tea	Crisp toast, spread when cold and split into sandwiches with sieved egg or soft cheese, or with honey or jelly-type jam Plain cake or biscuit Weak tea
Supper	As lunch, with weak coffee afterwards, if desired
Evening	Small milky drink Slices of banana or yam

Diet for general use with Crohn's disease

When the symptoms are not troublesome or you are in complete remission, the guiding principle is high protein and low fat.
  Points to note:

1 Protein is the build-and-repair food. Twice a day have a protein meal, with meat, fish, egg or cheese as the main ingredient for at least one of them. For the other you may choose vegetable proteins with pulses and grains, Quark and Quorn, nuts. Disadvantages of vegetarian foods are that they do not supply vitamin B12 (essential) and it is difficult to take in enough calories, especially since you cannot have extra fat.
2 Once or twice a week have fish, preferably salmon, sardine, herring, tuna or mackerel – or shark.
3 Carbohydrates, the energy foods, supply the bulk of your diet, but beware of highly purified sugar, highly refined flour products or polished rice. Alcohol counts as sugar.
4 Fats and oils: fish oil from the fatty fish above is especially beneficial in Crohn's, but be sparing with other fats.
5 Fibre is another food that is particularly useful in Crohn's. Choose, by trial and error, which type is least likely to give you excess gas, especially if you have a stoma. Eat plenty of fruits and vegetables, either raw or nearly so. Pick wholemeal bread, pasta and spaghetti.
6 If you must cook, microwave, steam, grill or bake in foil.
7 *Rarely* have a burger, luncheon meat, sausages, processed ham, cakes, biscuits, ice cream or pizza.
8 Remember you are trying to maintain or increase your weight.

High protein, low fat general purpose diet

On waking   Tea or fruit juice

Breakfast   Fruit juice (optional)
             Cereal with fresh or stewed fruit
             Egg, sardine, slice of cheese or ham, tomato
             Wholemeal toast with spread, honey or
               marmalade
             Coffee, tea or low fat chocolate

Mid-morning Drink as above and/or piece of fruit

119

Lunch	Meat, fish, egg or cheese with salad or two vegetables, or baked potato or wholemeal bread sandwich filled with any of the above, plus a side salad
	or
	Vegetable soup with wholemeal bread, if there is protein at two other meals
	Fresh or stewed fruit or baked apple with yogurt, fruit fool, rice pudding and fruit, upside-down cake
	Herb tea, fruit drink or mineral water
	Coffee – not too often in the day or too strong
Tea	Sandwich, or oatcake and cheese or Marmite
	Fresh fruit
	Drink as above
Supper	Soup (optional)
	Meat, fish, egg or cheese dish, plus two vegetables as well as potatoes, brown rice, wholemeal roll or pasta
	Fresh fruit, cheese and biscuits or yogurt
	Glass of wine, preferably white
	Herb tea, coffee or tea
Evening	Small hot drink, and a piece of fruit or biscuit if you wish

Follow this with enough sleep to wake refreshed.

Don't let yourself feel restricted by these suggestions – try as many as possible from the huge variety of fruits and vegetables available in both supermarkets and village stores these days, from all the corners of the earth. Sample all the different types of bread and forms of pasta. Only with the serious protein foods need you ring the changes more conservatively.

Bon appetit – live well!

11

Feeling and coping: the psychological aspects

The moment of truth – the diagnosis of Crohn's disease is a watershed in your life. Nothing will ever be quite the same. It may hit you in one of three ways:

- Shock and disbelief – suddenly you are a person with a serious disorder.
- Heart-sinking confirmation of what you had suspected for some time: the only difference is that now it has a label.
- Relief at sharing the problem and having an ally in dealing with it.

After the initial impact, an avalanche of thoughts and questions comes tumbling into your mind:

- Why me? Is it anything I've done?
- It isn't fair.
- What will happen next? Will I get better? Could I die?
- What will happen to my job? How much time off will I need?
- Will my physical status interfere with what I do?
- What will the treatment be like? Is it painful? Might I have to have an operation? (This is the point when horrific stories come to mind, about a great-uncle or someone's friend who had a bowel problem which might have been Crohn's.)
- How will the family react? What shall I tell them?
- How will the most important person in my life feel about my having a nasty illness? Will it wreck the relationship?
- What will it do to my sex life? If a man, will I be impotent? If a woman, will I still be attractive? Would I be able to have a baby?
- Suppose I have to rush to the loo at a crucial time?
- What will my friends think? How shall I explain?

Worst of all is the knock to your self-confidence, especially if you had always taken your body and its efficient functioning as read. There is nothing dignified, let alone romantic, about an illness that affects the bowels. All those crude sayings about 'arseholes', 'shit' and 'up yours' jump out at you – from the television, a book or a conversation overheard.

You may feel you are losing control, not only of your bowels but of your life. This feeling is only temporary, while you find the best way, for you, of getting to grips with the situation. There are several well-worn methods of coping with adversity:

1 Forced optimism – denying that there is anything seriously wrong. 'Just a touch of gastric flu', you say, 'I'm all right in myself', 'It's nothing to fuss about' – although you are feeling dreadful. The ploy can be useful to carry you through the first shock, while your mind adjusts to the reality. The danger is that it may lead you into refusing to have the treatment you need.

2 The opposite – passive acceptance and stoicism, which amount to pessimism. 'What will be, will be', 'It's no good fighting against it', or even, 'It's God's will'. This is definitely the worst attitude to any problem. You are programming yourself for invalidism.

3 Anger and resentment – this is better than Number 2, but you are wasting your energy. There is nothing constructive about ill-feeling and it is a rebuff to the army of people – friends, loved ones, professionals and acquaintances – who want to give you their support, if you let them.

4 Leaving the effort, the decisions and the responsibility to others, allowing yourself to become dependent. That scenario gives you nothing to plan, nothing more inspiring to look forward to than lunch.

5 Taking on the real enemy – the illness – with all the courage and determination you can muster. You know this makes most sense. Decide now that you are going to do whatever it takes to beat Crohn's disease, and you are not going to let it rob you of what you most value in life. This may be slightly different now, so take time to assess it:

- Relationships with the people who matter to you.
- Contributing to the general good, and specifically to the happiness of your particular people. This does wonders for your feeling of self-worth.
- Independence combined with graceful acceptance of help, including not being too proud to ask when you need it. People love to be a help.
- Making *new* friends and developing *new* interests. Treat life as an escalator.

What sort of people get Crohn's disease?

The smart answer is the unlucky ones. They are in every job or profession – music, accountancy, medicine, catering, earning £9,000 or £90,000. If people are alike in being susceptible to the same bug or illness, there is a theory that they may be similar psychologically. Each of us is a unique, irreplaceable individual, but nevertheless people with Crohn's are more likely than average to be reliable and responsible, but not bossy – good colleagues to work with or to have as friends. A common trait is self-control, not complaining until they absolutely have to and bottling up their feelings.

People with Crohn's are not typically the sort to throw their arms round you when they are happy, or weep on your shoulder when they feel bad. They tend to dislike fuss and conflict and prefer to avoid confrontation.

This may not be you at all. If you have an easy, relaxed attitude towards life and are a natural communicator, be glad. If, on the other hand, you are loath to display your feelings even when there is something on your mind as momentous as having Crohn's, other people will not guess what you are going through. Overcome your inhibitions and tell them of your anxiety, dismay and sense of unfairness, or simply ask questions, and it will relieve the tension. Dammed up emotions make pains and cramps worse, and unrelieved anxiety brings on diarrhoea. Negative emotions act directly on your immune system, suppressing it. So, on a purely practical, physical basis, you need to off-load the feelings that can disable your body's defences.

Communication is the key

You are not unusual if you find it difficult talking with doctors and nurses, especially doctors, finding out what you want to know, and telling them how you feel. More than 70 per cent of people find it a problem, and the chief killer of a useful exchange is that you are afraid they will think you are silly. They are not unsympathetic, but often they are embarrassed because they have not got the answers. Common difficulties are:

- Not remembering afterwards what the doctor said, particularly after the first, most important consultation, and then being too shy to ask. Maybe you did not ask a question because you were afraid of what the answer might be – and now you wish you had.
- Expressing your anxiety, depresssion or muddle, or that you are ashamed of the illness, illogically.
- Asking details about the treatment – what it will do and whether it has side-effects.
- Asking whether you are improving – medically.

If it is awkward talking with health professionals, it is no better with friends and relatives. What do you say when they tell you how much better you are looking, when you are feeling dreadful? Some of them visit you because of the illness but studiously talk about everything else, while others have an intrusive curiosity about the aspects you would rather not discuss. Some stay too long and wear you out ... but these are only pinpricks.

With the medical staff, be straightforward and determined – get your questions out or say what you feel at the first opportunity. With friends and relatives, tact is your strategy. The situation is strange for them too, but you need them. They are your emotional support system. The big benefit they confer is constant reassurance of your value as a person, well or ill. Expressing your feelings by telling them to other people takes the edge off the pain and puts things in perspective. It is good policy to spread the load by talking to as many of the people you know as possible. This way there is no danger, on the one hand, of burdening any one person, or, on the other, of hurting someone's feelings – 'Why didn't you tell me?'

People like to feel they are a help – and anyone who can make you laugh is worth their weight in gold.

Depression and anxiety

You are bound to feel unhappy and anxious some of the time. The understandable lowering of mood and haunting anxiety about the illness sometimes peaks into panicky feelings when a crisis threatens – how will you cope? When it actually happens, nine times out of ten you will rise to the occasion and do all the right things automatically. On the tenth time it will be taken out of your hands. The medics will know what to do.

Ralph
Ralph was a man who prided himself on never losing his cool. All through the ups and downs of his Crohn's, over the last eight years, he had managed to keep his sense of control. He discussed his medication and the dosage with the doctor, and understood his explanations of the pathology underlying the symptoms, and what the barium enema showed. Ralph decided against having a colonoscopy, although the gastroenterologist advised it. Ralph's disease was mainly in the colon and by care with his diet, regular prednisolone and will-power, he had managed to take hardly any time off work.

'Better than the youngsters', he would boast. He was now 58. It happened in March, when he was taking a brisk walk in a biting east wind. His blood pressure, which had been creeping up over the last few years, must have reacted to the cold and the exercise with a sudden surge. What Ralph noticed was the weird, warm feeling of blood pouring from his back passage. He had not the slightest control over it and he began to feel dizzy. He was frightened, a feeling he had never before admitted in himself, and was thankful to be bundled into an ambulance. From then on, until after the operation, he let other people take responsibility over decision-making.

It took him two or three months to get the hang of the ileostomy but much longer to come to terms with having lost his colon. Now, 18 months later, Ralph is back in control of his body, including its changed anatomy, his feelings and his job. He sees himself as something of an expert in Crohn's. The other bonus is that he and his wife have learned to talk about their feelings as well as the illness.

Clinical depression

Anxiety and depression in the everyday sense are endemic in Crohn's disease. Clinical depression and anxiety are something else. They are illnesses in their own right, and require specialist treatment. Depression as an illness not only drains your energy, it siphons off all hope and any possibility of happiness or of feeling anything at all for your nearest and dearest. Guilt pervades your mind, not for anything you have done, but just for being you. Even if you sleep, it brings no relief. Although it seems like a life sentence, you will emerge from this black hole – but treatment is essential if it is not to go on for months.

Esther
Esther was devastated to find that she had Crohn's disease. Her boyfriend took off when she looked like being a drag, and this did not help, especially as she had fallen out with her parents over him. Esther was 17 and no more moody than most teenagers. Her mother had been through mild postnatal depression after Esther was born, but otherwise there was no history of psychiatric illness in the family. Her parents were worried about the Crohn's, but not greatly concerned about what they called 'the grumps'.

Esther had been put on a fairly high dose of prednisolone to damp down the pain and diarrhoea initially, and this may have been partly responsible for the low, negative mood which now engulfed her. She would not eat, did not want to talk and spent most of the day sitting and staring. She could not be bothered to put on any make-up or care what clothes she wore. She blamed herself for the illness – which was not at all like her usual self. She felt worse as the day wore on and went to bed early to escape, but found she could not sleep.

Esther had a clinical depression. The counsellor attached to the surgery could do nothing to lift her mood. Esther needed the full antidepressant package, starting with seven weeks of intensive treatment with medication and cognitive therapy. She continued with the latter while the medication was reduced, but not stopped, for another five months, and she was able to go back to college part-way through. Maintenance treatment with medicines and discussion sessions, at first on a monthly basis, then two-monthly, went on for the rest of the year. The Crohn's symptoms had also come under control, now with non-steroid drugs. By the time Esther was through with the psychiatric treatment, like other sufferers from clinical depression, there had been plenty of opportunities to discuss and work through the stresses which had built up.

Cognitive psychotherapy without medication can be effective in depression but may require more expert therapist time than the NHS can afford. This is a talking treatment in which you are guided, logically, into understanding your mental state and getting rid of the harmful automatic thoughts and reactions which are maintaining the depression.

Anxiety states

Anxiety states are acutely distressing, but they do not carry the deadly depressive sense of guilt and hopelessness, where there is a risk of getting so bad that suicide seems an option. Medication, including some of the modern, post-Prozac antidepressants, may also help in anxiety, but it is more a matter for constructive discussion with a psychologist, and active involvement in overcoming whatever you fear.

Both depression and anxiety are liable to come back if there is a sudden down-turn in your physical state, or some other blow, or a slow build of stress – for instance at work. No one can keep stress out of their life long term. The trick is to manage it.

One big stressful event is having an operation involving a colostomy or ileostomy. This is a major life-event, and you must allow time for your body, and even more important, your mind, to adjust, for there to be harmonious co-operation between the two. The practical aspects are dealt with in Chapter 9, but being at peace with yourself with a changed body can be hard to achieve. A firm foundation lies in building good relationships – at home, in the outside world, at work. If they were not brilliant before, now is an opportunity, as a new, mended person, to put that right.

People are your lifeline, even when your instinct tells you to shut yourself away. Time on your own – to think – is bad for you, and although you need adequate sleep (six to eight hours) too much time in bed will lower your mood. Since your stoma is now part of you, you may as well start living to your full potential with it. Of course there will be days when you are fed up, down or worried, but live through these, pick yourself up and carry on. This is the achievement to be proud of.

While depression and anxiety can be disabling illnesses in themselves, often they are part of Crohn's. You need to evolve ploys to cushion yourself against them. Here are some which work for me:

- Keeping friendships in good repair.
- A well-developed habit of sharing your feelings and ideas when they are fresh, not only with established friends, but new acquaintances, too. Not everybody will want to know the physical details about your bowels, but they can all relate to feelings of worry or sadness – or what you look forward to or hope for. Day-to-day chit-chat is safer and better than popping Valium, and it relaxes your mind and body just as effectively.
- Exercise both stimulates and relaxes you, whether it is a session in the gym or a pool, or simply a half-hour walk.
- Exchanging affection with a dog or a cat is known to boost the immune system and promote healing, but better still must be sharing love with your chosen ones.

12
The future

Richard Quain, writing on chronic inflammation of the intestines in 1885, remarked what a 'debilitating and wearying' condition it was – and, at that time, invariably fatal. The methods of examination when the abdomen was 'the seat of the mischief' were simple:

- Inspection of the size and shape of the abdomen.
- Inserting a finger into the back passage, or blowing air into it, though for what purpose is unclear.
- Examination of the motions with the naked eye.

Treatment was similarly limited:

- quinine
- iron
- sea air
- removal of mental worry

Fifty years later Burrill Crohn suggested that 'his' disease might be caused by some species of mycobacterium, similar to the one responsible for tuberculosis. Research into Crohn's disease ran round in circles for another half century vainly trying to find the bug. Meanwhile DNA was discovered and we had entered the technological age.

In 1989 Professor Joseph Kirsner of Chicago was confidently forecasting the use of DNA probes to identify different species of micro-organisms, although he was bemoaning the lack of success in linking any one of them, convincingly, with Crohn's. The prevalence of the disease was already accelerating (there are now 500,000 cases in the USA) and although the areas most affected were in Western Europe and North America, it appeared to have a worldwide distribution. Kirsner knew of cases in Algeria, Bagwanath and among the Chinese in Canada. He thought that autoimmunity was a key cause, possibly through proteins from viruses or bacteria becoming incorporated into the lining cells of the gut. He had hopes of a vaccine being developed against all autoimmune disease. This has not yet happened.

The mechanism by which stress is implicated in Crohn's in both humans and cows still needs investigating, and also how cigarettes fit in. Pharmaceutical research has produced ever more effective medicines –

each with its potential for side-effects. Cyclosporin, used in difficult cases of Crohn's, is one such. The first report of serious effects on the brain and nervous system with this drug came out in the *British Medical Journal* in April 1999. It seems that the danger occurs when cyclosporin is used in conjunction with some other medicines, including prednisolone and methotrexate. The first is used frequently in Crohn's, the latter occasionally.

On the surgical front, stricturoplasty, a simple, localized operation, has become the standard for relieving intestinal obstruction or the threat of it, and microtechnical instruments are constantly being improved. Another advance is in cancer surveillance. Cancer is a complication that can arise in long-term Crohn's disease. There are now techniques for detecting the early changes, before an actual cancer develops, in the same way as a cervical smear.

In the early 1990s, Professor J. Hermon-Taylor and his team from St George's Hospital, London, entered the arena with outstanding zeal for their mycobacterium theory of the cause of Crohn's. Since 1913, even before Crohn published his work, something akin to mycobacterium tuberculosis was suspected of being responsible for inflammation of the intestines in humans as well as cows. They could not see it but they called it mycobacterium paratuberculosis (Mptb). We now believe that this bug can live in the soil, in rivers and on plants, and that cows can harbour Mptb without being ill. Some of them, however, develop the Crohn's-like illness, Johne's disease. Modern, intensive milk-production methods may serve to concentrate these bacteria in certain places.

Two major problems bedevilling research have been, first, the difficulty in identifying Mptb from the many other micro-organisms in cow-pats and human motions, and second, growing it in culture. Now the polymerase chain reaction (PCR) in combination with increasingly refined DNA probes can identify Mptb, even in small quantities, though not yet as a routine procedure. A tiresome stumbling block remains – the finicky nature of Mptb, taking many months to grow in culture, if at all.

Food scares are commonplace and Mptb has provided two. In 1996 Professor Hermon-Taylor suggested that Mptb in milk and milk products could infect people and cause Crohn's disease. Nothing much was done about this. More recently, he indicated that drinking water might also be a vehicle for Mptb. Cattle slurry could possibly be contaminating water supplies. This view was aired on Channel 4 News in April 1999. Apparently some of these bacteria can survive pasteurization, in the case of milk, and the water purification process. This, of course, does not prove that taking in some Mptb causes Crohn's in normal circumstances. We all swallow millions of germs in our daily lives.

However, one study shows that more of the people with Crohn's have Mptb in their intestines than those without Crohn's, including sufferers from ulcerative colitis, which it so much resembles. If Mptb is a major cause of Crohn's disease, it should be curable with antimycobacterial antibiotics, such as azithromycin or clarithromycin. These and other drugs are currently the subject of trials, but there has been no breakthrough. Any beneficial effects have been slow to develop and have not been dramatic.

Professor Hermon-Taylor's theories are attractive and it may well be the Mptb is heavily implicated in a fair proportion of cases, but it cannot be the sole cause of the disease. The connection with ulcerative colitis, including what appears to be a genetic link, yet the marked differences between the two illnesses, remains unexplained. Or why you are more likely to develop Crohn's if you have a brother or sister with the disease than a parent.

Those who work in the field of Crohn's, and know most about it, are divided over Professor Hermon-Taylor's ideas. The National Association for Colitis and Crohn's disease (NACC) is highly sceptical. The good thing is that the government is now pledged to investigate the whole matter 'extremely seriously'.

What causes Crohn's disease? Perhaps they will find the answer.

Useful addresses

United Kingdom

National Association for Colitis and Crohn's disease (NACC)
PO Box 205
St Albans
Herts AL1 5HH
Tel: 01727 844296
http://www.nacc.org.uk/contact.htm

Crohn's in Childhood Research Association (CICRA)
356 West Barnes Lane
Motspur Park
Surrey KT3 6NB
Tel: 0208 949 6209

Teens with Crohn's Disease Website
http://pages.prodigy.com/teencron/

British Colostomy Association
15 Station Road
Reading
Berks RG1 1LG
Freephone 0800 328 4257

The Ileostomy and Internal Pouch Support Group
PO Box 123
Scunthorpe
North Lincs DN15 9YW
Tel: 01724 844296
http://www.ileostomypouch.demon.co.uk

National Ankylosing Spondylitis Society (NASS)
PO Box 179
Mayfield
East Sussex TN40 6ZL
Tel: 01435 873527
http://web.ukonline.co.uk/nass/

Europe

European Foundation of Crohn's and Ulcerative Colitis Associations (EFFCA)
Eighteen associations throughout Europe
Secretariat
Beukenlaan 3
4356 HJ Oostkapelle
The Netherlands
Tel: 31 (0) 118 58 60 73
http://www.nacc.org.uk/effca/efcmem.htm

United States of America

Crohn's and Colitis Foundation of America, Inc. (CCFA)
386 Park Avenue South
17th floor
New York
NY10016–8804
USA
Tel: (212) 685 3440
    (800) 932 2423
http://www.ccfa.org/

Intestinal Disease Foundation
1323 Forbes Avenue
Suite 200
Pittsburg
PA15219
USA
Tel: (412) 261 5888

The Pediatric Crohn's and Colitis Association
PO Box 18
Newton
MA02168–0002
USA
Tel: (617) 290 0902

Canada

Crohn's and Colitis Foundation of Canada (CCFC)
21 St Clair Avenue East
Suite 301
Toronto
Ontario
Canada M4T 1L9
Tel: (416) 920 5035 Ext. 21
www.ccfc.ca

Australia

Australian Crohn's and Colitis Association Inc (ACCA)
PO Box 201
Mooroolbark
Victoria 3138
Australia
Tel: 61 3 9276 9914
Email: acca@ozramp.net.au

Australian Crohn's and Colitis Association (Qld) Inc (ACCAQ)
PO Box 548
Maleny
Queensland 4552
Australia
Tel: 61 7 5494 2149
http://www.accaq.org.au

South Australia Crohn's and Colitis Association Inc (SACCA)
PO Box 3153
Rundle Mail
Adelaide
SA 5000
Australia
Tel: 61 8 8449 4357
http://www.accaq.org.au/text/affiliates/acca.htm

USEFUL ADDRESSES

New Zealand

Crohn's and Colitis Support Group Inc (CCSG)
PO Box 24–171
Royal Oak
Auckland
New Zealand
Tel: 64 9 6367228
http://home.clear.net.nz/pages/ccsg/clearhome.html

Index

135

INDEX

stomach 7–8; elective surgery 73; nausea and vomiting 23
stricturoplasty 73, 75
sulphasalazine (salazopyrin) 25, 64–5, 68
surgery: elective 71–7, 81–2; emergencies 60–71, 80–1; post-operative diet 103; preparation 71–3, 82–3

tiredness 103
tomatoes 95
town versus country 12–13
toxic colitis 77–8, 81
toxic megacolon 70, 78, 81
travel 89–90

ultrasound 53–4
urinary system 46–7, 74

vaginal fistulas 74
vitamins and minerals 26–7; anaemia 42–4; clotting 69–70; malabsorption 55–6; mineral-providing foods 110–12; undernutrition 103–4; vitamin-providing foods 104–10

wheat 94–5
work 90

X-rays: barium enema 51, 82–3; barium meal 50; CT scanning 52, 83; enteroclysis 50–1; ultrasound 83

yeast 95